SPORTS SLUMP BUSTING

10 Steps To Mental Toughness And Peak Performance

Alan S. Goldberg

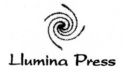

Llumina Press

D1531087

© 2005 Alan S. Goldberg

All rights reserved. No part of this publication may be reproduced or transmitted in any form or by any means electronic or mechanical, including photocopy, recording, or any information storage and retrieval system, without permission in writing from both the copyright owner and the publisher.

Requests for permission to make copies of any part of this work should be mailed to Permissions Department, Llumina Press, PO Box 772246, Coral Springs, FL 33077-2246

ISBN: 1-59526-101-X

Printed in the United States of America by Llumina Press

Library of Congress Control Number: 2005926663

To the child within

There's a child inside of you who holds the key to your greatest dreams. While he may be temporarily frightened by other people and events, he refuses to let go of those dreams. He tugs at your leg for attention. He whines for you to notice him. He whispers in your ear of all that you can be. Sometimes you'd just like him to go away with all that silliness. No such luck. He's too persistent. He's determined to get noticed. He refuses to give up. You've tried to talk some reason into him, but thankfully he won't listen. Others have told him the "facts" and the limits on what's possible. He's not interested in their "impossibles." He does not understand "can't." He doesn't care if others laugh at his dreams, as long as you don't. He wants you to consider the possibilities. He wants to show you what he can do. He will not quit until he's gotten your attention. His spirit can't be broken. He refuses to stay down. His resiliency is awe inspiring. His enthusiasm is refreshing and boundless. Harness that child within. Learn to listen to him. Let him guide you to your dreams.

After two weeks of watching the 1996 Atlanta Olympic Games on TV, my daughter Julee announced to us that *she* wanted to become an Olympian in swimming and gymnastics. She had no way of knowing that the athletes competing in Atlanta had begun their Olympic quests many years ago with this same kind of childlike pronouncement. Julee is listening to that child inside of her. She is in close contact with her. How about you? Are you *really* listening?

CONTENTS

Preface
vi

Acknowledgments
viii

Introduction
10 Steps From the Pits to the Peak
1

Step 1
Ruling Out Nonmental Causes
9

Step 2
Establishing Self-Control
23

Step 3
Developing a Championship Focus
45

Step 4
Dealing With Your Fears
75

Step 5
Expecting Success
99

Step 6
Developing Positive Images
131

Step 7
Setting Slump-Busting Goals
165

Step 8
Building Self-Confidence
199

Step 9
Becoming Mentally Tough
219

Step 10
Insuring Against Future Slumps
241

Appendix
Relaxation Exercises
261

Notes
267

Bibliography
269

Index
271

About the Author
277

PREFACE

As a junior tennis player, I intuitively took advantage of my greatest strength, the mental side of my game. Not a physically overpowering athlete, I wore down even stronger and more talented opponents with relentlessness and tenacity. I became fascinated by the power of the mind to either enhance or sabotage performance. Twelve years ago this fascination intensified as I began to work with athletes who were struggling with specific performance blocks: a diver immobilized by fears who was suddenly unable to execute a dive that she had done perfectly hundreds of times; a gymnast blocked for over a year on a back handspring on the beam after watching a teammate get hurt on the same skill; and a 1,000-yard-a-season college running back who, in his senior year, could no longer find the hole.

As I tried to help these athletes solve their problems, I realized that similar, inexplicable, and repeated performance difficulties also stalked teams: a college basketball team that had lost 11 games in a row, over half the losses to weaker teams; a defending conference-champion football team that lost the first five games of its season, despite the fact that the team was even stronger than the previous year; a high school soccer team that had a long history of losing in the playoffs to teams they had crushed during the regular season; and finally, and painfully, my beloved Red Sox, who always seem to manage a late-season swoon every fall to drop out of contention.

The 10-step slump-busting model emerged from my work with and observation of these athletes and teams. Almost all athletes struggle with poor performances at one time or another. Some emerge from these struggles quickly and with renewed strength. Those are the athletes with a psychic resiliency or "mental toughness." Other athletes, however, become mired in these poor performances. Their inability to let go mentally of their frustrations and disappointments makes them vulnerable to more failures.

Most slumps start this way in the athletes' minds. Despite the fact that the solution to their performance problem is in their heads, slumping athletes either don't look there, or if they do, they don't know what to do with what they find. Consequently, slumps leave them feeling out of control and powerless. These feelings, in turn, erode an already shaky self-confidence and fuel the slump cycle.

Sports Slump Busting was written to help you, the athlete, get back in control. Its purpose is to provide you with the means—a 10-step model—to get your performance back on track. Whether you're struggling at the plate, consistently fall apart in the big competitions, are immobilized by a performance fear, or are overwhelmed with frustration because your efforts in practice are not paying off at crunch time, *Sports Slump Busting* will help you get your mind and body working together again. It is a practical guidebook for slump busting and developing mental toughness.

Sports Slump Busting will be useful to amateur and professional athletes alike across all sports. It is a powerful tool *if used properly*. The book includes numerous questionnaires and exercises that will help you not only understand your performance difficulties, but also develop the ability to positively turn them around. In other words, plan on *doing* the book while you read it. Take ample time to think about and complete each exercise.

Sports Slump Busting is also an important tool for coaches. It will help coaches better understand the causes of slumps and provides practical strategies for breaking and avoiding slumps. *Sports Slump Busting* will also provide coaches with the basics of mental toughness and stimulate ideas about how these can be integrated into their basic coaching repertoire. The book will help coaches more effectively intervene with their athletes or team struggling with repeated performance problems.

For most parents of competitive athletes, performance slumps are difficult to understand. Consequently, well-meaning parents can say or do things that only seem to worsen the problems. *Sports Slump Busting* will help these parents better understand the causes of slumps and what they can do to help their child get back on track.

Although it directly deals with the topic of blocks and slumps, *Sports Slump Busting* is really a book about peak performance and winning. It provides the mental techniques and skills necessary to become a mentally tough peak performer, regardless of the sport. Therefore, this book is more than a crisis intervention tool. *Sports Slump Busting* is a book about "mental fitness" that deals with a negative topic, slumps, in a positive, solutions-oriented way. While I have included numerous examples of athletes besieged by performance difficulties, I have also highlighted many positive and inspiring examples of professional and amateur athletes who have stood their ground against the slump monster and won.

While slumps and blocks will always be part of athletic performance, *Sports Slump Busting* will provide you with the mental toughness tools to keep these normal, frustrating experiences brief and infrequent. Because it teaches mental toughness skills and highlights the dynamics of performance blocks and the kinds of thinking from which they arise, *Sports Slump Busting* will become your insurance policy against future slumps.

While other mental-toughness books on the market briefly address the topic of slumps, none provide such practical, in-depth coverage of this frustrating performance malady as *Sports Slump Busting*. With its unique 10-step slump-busting model and positive emphasis, *Sports Slump Busting* is sure to become an important piece of equipment for the athlete and coach interested in winning and peak performance.

ACKNOWLEDGMENTS

There are many people I'd like to sincerely thank who made this book possible: my colleagues, Dr. Rob Gilbert, for being an unlimited and constant source of ideas and inspiration, and Pete Greider, for his support and willingness to be a sounding board; Julia Demmin, for her encouragement, help in editing, and unconditional belief in me; my wife and best friend, Renee Hill, for her patience, love, and support, which allowed me to give free reign to my creativity; my daughters Sara and Julee, for bringing their light into my life and providing me with ample opportunities to play; Judy Wolfson, a friend, for her willingness to read the manuscript and her enthusiasm for the project.

Special thanks go to the coaches and athletes who have helped me develop my slump-busting approach over the years: coaches Richard Quick, Jeffrey Pill, David Caster, Andy Wedaman, and Bill Boomer, for their stories and ideas; and special appreciation to the hundreds of athletes who have trusted me enough to teach me about their sports and share with me their frustrations and struggles.

Thanks also to Stephen and Carol Lankton and John Edgette for their Ericksonian Hypnosis training, which has had a profound influence in shaping my work with the slumping or stuck athlete.

I would also like to thank the people at Human Kinetics who have helped me make this book a reality, especially Julie Marx, Jacqueline Blakley, and Ted Miller for their wonderful feedback and great ideas.

INTRODUCTION

10 STEPS FROM THE PITS TO THE PEAK

If you compete in sports long enough, sooner or later you'll have the rare pleasure of experiencing one of those truly magical moments. As your mind and body come together in perfect harmony, you temporarily slip into a zone of performance that we usually think is just reserved for superstars. Suddenly, you're Michael Jordan, shooting out of your mind, draining one long jumper after another and pulling off moves that defy gravity and the seeming limits of human ability. Or maybe you're transformed into Tiger Woods, leaving your opponents in the dust as you drop yet another birdie putt to open a dominating lead. Or you find yourself in Steffi Graf's shoes on center court, hitting one amazing shot after another to beat a skilled and determined opponent.

When athletes enter the so-called "zone," they have that almost mystical experience that makes the sacrifices and long, painful hours of training all worthwhile. There's nothing more personally satisfying than having everything effortlessly come together for you. Your muscles instantly respond as programmed with powerful, fluid movements. Your senses are heightened and precise as you react perfectly to every situation without conscious thought or effort. For that brief moment, you're in harmony with the universe, and the gods of peak performance are smiling on you.

Unfortunately, peak performance and the zone are not always waiting for you when you suit up. All too often you go out to play with great expectations and find that your mind and body are totally out of sync that day. You hope to walk on water but instead find yourself moving in slow motion under ten feet of the wet stuff, feeling uncomfortable and uncoordinated. It's as if the connection between your brain and muscles has short-circuited. You have two left feet, stone fingers, and a concrete elbow all at the worst possible time. Your bases-loaded, game-on-the-line opportunity ends in a huge whiff, your fourth that day. You just don't seem to have that all-important "feel" before the competition. You've misplaced your jump shot and can't buy a basket. Although you shot an amazing eight under par for the front nine yesterday, today with uncanny accuracy you find every tree, bunker, and impossible lie on the same course for a 15 over.

Like the good ones, these bad performances are a normal part of sports. No one is at his or her best all the time. There are always peaks and valleys in how you feel and perform. However, sometimes you or your team may get lost in one of these valleys and can't seem to find your way out. Days, weeks, and even months go by, yet you remain stuck in subpar play. You may put together a string of poor performances, losing several contests in a row, or routinely collapse at the last minute in a match to snatch defeat from the jaws of victory. Or suddenly you may "lose" a skill that you've had forever, and no matter where you look or how hard you try, you just can't get it back. When these poor performances move into your game, and like an unwanted house guest, refuse to leave, you are in a slump.

While it seems that the best athletes are immune to slumps, this is not the case. Even the great ones occasionally stumble. Tennis legend Martina Navratilova rarely struggled when in her prime, yet early in her career, she was considered by many to be mentally undisciplined and a "head case," frequently losing matches to less-talented players. Sadaharu Oh, the "Japanese Babe Ruth" and one of the greatest hitters of all time, went into a hitting slump that lasted for almost two years.

Sometimes slumps become so bad that they can drive an athlete out of the sport. Former New York Mets starting catcher Mackey Sasser lost his job because of a sudden inability to throw the ball back to the pitcher. Sasser felt compelled to pump the ball two or three times into his glove before lobbing it back to the mound. Base runners were then able to time Sasser's feeble return tosses and make delayed steals. Similarly, former Dodger second baseman Steve Sax suddenly found that he could no longer throw the ball accurately during routine plays, a mysterious slump-like affliction that later became known around the league as the "Steve Sax disease."

Occasionally, a team's or athlete's slump can clearly be traced to technical or mechanical problems. The athlete may be unknowingly using faulty technique. Physical strength or flexibility may be underdeveloped. Perhaps the athlete lacks adequate speed or the team is thin on offensive talent. Slumps can even get their start from a previous injury.

Frequently, however, repeated performance problems seem to mysteriously emerge out of thin air. Like the flu, they can spread quickly through the athlete's repertoire of skills, affecting every aspect of his performance and sapping his self-confidence. On a team, one player's slump can "infect" almost everyone around her. When this happens, the results can be devastating.

The 1995 California Angels are a painful example of a contagious slump. In mid-August, they were 64–38 and running away with the American

League West, leading the majors in runs scored, and being hailed as the best team in the 35-year history of the franchise. Then they went into a roller-coaster slide that eliminated them from playoff contention and earned them the ignominious record for the fastest disappearance of a 10 1/2 game lead (August 16–September 20) in this century.

How could this have happened with such a talented team? Some people think the California hitting and pitching slumped at the same time, perhaps triggered by injuries to key players and aggravated by the inexperience of their young squad. For the Angels and so many other athletes and teams, the questions of *how* a slump starts and *why* it continues remain unanswered. Even more important, how to *break free* from the slump's nasty clutches remains a mystery not easily solved.

Perhaps the main reason for a slump's enduring nature is that most slumps seem to be directly related to the athlete's psyche or "mental game," an area traditionally considered off-limits by most coaches. Many coaches believe that not only are the athletes' inner workings beyond their expertise, but also "messing with their heads" could cause serious mental problems. As a result, coaches have adopted a hands-off approach and simply label athletes stuck in slumps as "head cases," a label that only reinforces the athletes' already low self-confidence and contributes to their performance problems.

The real story about slumps, however, is that most are neither mysterious nor a result of an athlete's "mental weaknesses." Instead, slumps are simply a result of the athlete's mind and body being out of sync. Rather than working together, the athlete's head is getting in the way of body and muscle memory.

The majority of slumps follow a predictable cycle that can be easily understood and interrupted. The cycle usually starts after a bad performance or two touches off negativity, self-doubts, and worries in the athletes' minds. Going into the next competition, the athletes are preoccupied with these past failures and concerned that they may repeat them. Consequently, they have the wrong focus of concentration and try to overcontrol the present performance. Because they are too tense and are not paying attention to the cues that would enable them to do their best, they fail again. One more failure further erodes their confidence and continues to distract them from what's important. In this way, the athletes set in motion a negative cycle in their minds that seems to take on a life of its own.

Sports Slump Busting was written to unravel the slump mystery and provide coaches and athletes with clear and practical answers to their numerous questions about repetitive performance problems: Where do slumps come from? Why are they so infectious? Is there anything I can do to avoid catching one? And, most important, how do I bust out of a slump?

Through my work with hundreds of slumping athletes and teams across a wide variety of sports, I have put together an effective 10-step slump-busting program that is both preventative and corrective. First, it will help you, the athlete or coach, identify the mental mistakes, warning signs, and mind-set that pull an athlete or team into a slump. Second, it provides a set of mental skills and strategies that return athletes to optimal performance and develop and reinforce mental toughness.

The Principles of Peak Performance

Few slumping athletes realize that the road from the pits to the peak starts in their past peak performances. For example, in 1968 three-time Olympic gold medal discus thrower Al Oerter was competing in an amazing fourth Olympics. After his next-to-last throw, Oerter found himself out of medal contention and throwing poorly. In the few minutes that remained before his final attempt, Oerter went off by himself and began to systematically think about his last Olympics when he had won a gold medal and set a world record. As he had practiced many times before, he mentally reviewed, in detail, all the sights, sounds, kinesthetic (muscle) feelings, and emotions from that 1964 medal-winning performance in Tokyo. Having recaptured these "winning feelings," Oerter then, with his last toss, won the gold an unprecedented fourth time!

How could Oerter go from the pits to the peak so quickly? Was there something magical about this mental reviewing of a past great performance? If so, can you learn to duplicate Oerter's magic act?

As Oerter demonstrated, the key to slump busting lies within your past great performances and the mind-set that you carried *into* and *through* those experiences. Over the years, hundreds of athletes and teams at the top of their games have taught me that, when you're at your best, seven mental characteristics are *always* present. Not surprisingly, these seven characteristics are conspicuously absent when you're caught in the clutches of a slump. If you can learn to mix the following seven principles into your mental game as you perform, you'll be well on your way to busting that slump and consistently turning out one great performance after another.

Principle #1—Passion and Fun

You must be passionate about your sport. You must be excited about putting it all on the line and being pushed to your limits by the competition. You must enjoy the struggle, the challenge, the ups and downs, and everything about training and competing. This kind of passion fuels you to become a champion. If you go into a performance having fun, then you will do your best. Athletes who wait until they win before they can enjoy themselves don't do either, because they have it backward! Passion comes first; then peak performance.

Principle #2—High Self-Confidence

How you perform is always dictated by your level of confidence. Average athletes or teams with above-average confidence will consistently perform above their abilities. Confidence is that magical catalyst that converts those long hours of training, your physical skills, and your conditioning into successful execution under pressure. Self-confidence helps you face off against adversity, setbacks, or losses and come out on top and in control. Without self-confidence, a slump has fertile soil to take root and grow out of control.

Principle #3—Concentration on the Process of the Performance

Concentration is one of the keys to athletic excellence. What you focus on before and during your performance will determine your success or failure. To do your best, you must learn to concentrate on the *process* of the performance, not the *outcome*. Focusing on the process means that you focus your attention *on the action as it unfolds in the immediate moment*. Outcome thoughts like winning, losing, getting a hit, or scoring a goal usually interfere with doing your best and keep the slump cycle going.

Principle #4—Resilience

When you're really "on," thoughts of failure get no airtime. You have the ability to quickly rebound from mistakes, setbacks, and bad breaks. Should you stumble or get knocked down, you pop right back up, brush yourself off, and continue on as if nothing had happened. Mistakes immediately fade out of your mental picture as you keep yourself focused on what's important. Unlike the slumping athlete, you do not have an "inner statistician" keeping track of all your missed plays, defensive blunders, and embarrassing moments. Resilience is a mental skill of champions, and it can lift your performance to the next level.

Principle #5—A Sense of Challenge

When you're "in the groove," you respond automatically to an inner sense of purpose. You're on a mission and rise to the challenge presented by that mission. Whether it's a certain opponent, a "last chance" competition, or the need to prove yourself, you are *positively* motivated to stretch the limits of your ability. As you rise to this challenge, you are oblivious to all the negative consequences of failing. Slumping athletes are negatively motivated by threats, fears, and the "what-ifs," a mind-set that keeps them stuck.

Principle #6—A Nonthinking, Automatic Quality

One principle that is always present when you're "on" is a sort of mindlessness. You're not thinking; you're just doing. You're "on automatic," and all the appropriate movements seem to effortlessly flow out of you perfectly timed. You play out of your mind in this way because you trust your training and are into a let-it-happen mind-set. When Yogi Berra said, "a full mind is an empty bat," he was referring to the overthinking problems of the slumping athlete.

Principle #7—A Sense of Relaxation During the Performance

The previous six principles contribute to Principle #7, being relaxed throughout the performance. Being mentally and physically relaxed is a must for you to reach your peak. Being loose in this way allows for lightning-quick reflexes; perfect timing; and fluid, powerful execution of all your skills. Without this sense of mental and physical looseness, your movements are restricted and you can't perform to your potential.

Using *Sports Slump Busting*

In the 10-step slump-busting model that follows, I will show you how to find these seven peak-performance principles in yourself and then mix them together to more consistently produce the kind of athletic performance that will make you proud. This model will help you, as an athlete, to move your performance and attitude from the pits to the peak. And *Sports Slump Busting*'s 10 steps will provide coaches with a helpful framework for intervention with an individual athlete or the entire team. It will also give coaches the tools to teach athletes the basics of mental toughness.

What's the best way to use *Sports Slump Busting*? I've designed my 10-step model so that each step naturally flows from the preceding one. By starting in the beginning and working your way through the steps in order, you can develop a working understanding of the dynamics of slumps and how to bust out of them, developing in their place a solid foundation of mental toughness.

The steps in *Sports Slump Busting* have been distinctly separated, though most are interconnected and build on each other throughout the book. If you have a specific problem (e.g., lack of confidence, poor concentration, or fear), that you want to immediately address, you can go right to that step in the model. *Sports Slump Busting* was designed to support this kind of use by linking each step to other important and related steps. For example, regaining control (Step 2) directly affects all subsequent steps. The skill of concentration discussed in Step 3 provides the basis for regaining control (Step 2), overcoming fears (Step 4), developing confidence (Steps 5 and 8), becoming mentally tough (Step 9), and effectively handling pressure (Step 10). Step 7, "Setting Slump-Busting Goals," can be used to develop all the skills discussed in this book and is especially important in Step 4, "Dealing With Your Fears." Step 10 provides you with an insurance policy against future slumps and enables you to focus better (Step 3), constructively face your fears (Step 4), develop confidence (Step 5), successfully use slump-busting imagery, (Step 6), and develop mental toughness (Step 9).

Conclusion

A question frequently asked by the slumping athlete is, "How long will it take for me to end this slump?" The amount of time that it takes for you to bust that slump depends entirely on *you* and how much effort you're willing to put into this program. If you take each step one at a time and conscientiously do all the accompanying exercises, you may be surprised at how quickly you return to success. If you simply glance through the book without doing the exercises or practicing the slump-busting techniques, then you'll continue to experience frustration and may even drop your sport in despair.

As you read this book, it's important to keep in mind that *you already have the solution to the slump mystery inside of you.* One of the first things I say to a slumping athlete is, "I'm not going to teach you anything that you don't already know." You may have trouble trusting this statement, given your frustration and all your failed attempts to bust that slump. It's not that I'm a terminal optimist, either. It's just that I have watched many stuck athletes get unstuck by discovering what they already know. You will understand when you get the slump monkey off your back. Two things will happen after you've finished the book and successfully put the slump into the past. First, you'll be mentally tougher as a result of this process. Second, you'll discover that those bad days that are a normal part of every sport will be more fleeting in the future.

STEP 1

RULING OUT NONMENTAL CAUSES

"It's been broken for how long you say?
Six long months, 18 hours, and 1 day...
I gathered all my tools just in case
To unscrew, take apart, and replace.
I studied the problem long and then shrugged
In my great wisdom, I discovered it was unplugged."

Let's get right down to it. What's the very first step you must take to help bust that slump and restore your sanity? The road from the performance outhouse to the penthouse starts with a very simple understanding: Not all slumps are in your head. Sometimes a few very good reasons explain why your performances consistently give off a foul odor, and they may have nothing to do with your being a "head case."

Not all slumps are in your head.

Without question, peak performance is a by-product of your mind and body working together in perfect harmony. Most coaches and athletes would readily agree that the majority of slumps are a direct result of this harmony breaking down. Suddenly, instead of cooperating, your mind starts sabotaging your body. It may question your choice of strategies or technique, worry about your ability to execute successfully, or simply remind you at

9

the worst possible time of a recent failure. The result of all this mental interference is an athletic body that responds in a totally unrecognizable fashion.

However, not all slumps are caused by this mind-body battle. Sometimes your muscles just simply don't know what to do or how to do it. So when your moment finally comes—the crowd is hushed and the air is electric with excitement and anticipation—you short-circuit. Your timing may be off, your movements may lack the necessary flexibility, you may run out of gas, or you may not have the speed or strength to get the job done.

Four Key Areas
of Athletic Excellence

In every sport, athletic excellence and peak performance are made possible by the right combination of training in four key areas: two involve your body and two, your mind. These areas are the physical, technical, tactical, and mental. Although presented separately here, all are closely interrelated when you compete. You can't become a champion if you ignore any of these. You must work each one into your overall development and training as an athlete. If your performance mysteriously slides into the dumpster, before looking for mental causes first carefully explore the physical, technical, and tactical areas for slump-busting solutions.

If your performance slides into the dumpster, first explore the physical, technical, and tactical areas for solutions.

- **Physical**—This arena of training includes five basic components:
  1. Body strength (upper and lower)
  2. Agility—your ability to change directions quickly and efficiently
  3. Speed—how fast you can move from one point to another
  4. Flexibility—your ability to stretch a distance or rapidly change muscle length without damaging your muscles
  5. Endurance—the two energy systems in your body, anaerobic and aerobic

Building body strength requires skill repetition and weight training of the various muscle groups. Agility drills and repetitive training enhance your quickness and speed. To develop flexibility, systematically stretch the muscle groups relevant to your sport. Build anaerobic endurance with sprint and speed training in which your body doesn't get adequate oxygen to meet its needs. Develop aerobic endurance by practicing what 1996 Women's Olympic Swim Team coach Richard Quick described as "easy speed"—huge amounts of training that allow your body to meet the demands of your sport over the long haul.

• **Technical**—The technical arena of your sport refers to your mechanics and skill execution. It is, very simply, what you are able to do with your body—the form of your tennis stroke, the precision of your glovework, the accuracy of your shooting, or the fluidity of your skating and stick handling. You develop good technique under the close supervision of a knowledgeable coach through countless hours of practice and repetition.

• **Tactical**—The tactical part of your sport covers your knowledge of strategy and your ability to use this knowledge effectively by consistently making the right decisions under pressure. A soccer player's ability to anticipate a developing play and move into position without the ball or a football quarterback's skill in reading the opposing team's defense are good examples of tactical knowledge. Such knowledge is developed through good coaching, competitive experience, practice, studying videos, and reading.

• **Mental**—The mental arena includes your abilities to concentrate, handle pressure, rebound from mistakes and setbacks, and avoid dejection and intimidation, as well as your confidence level, motivation, and preparation for competition. The volleyball player who comes up with a huge dig when her team has its back against the wall or the basketball player who sinks the game-winning shot after missing his last five attempts are examples of athletes with strengths in this mental dimension. As with tactical acuity, mental toughness is developed through competitive experience, coaching, modeling of successful athletes, practice, and reading.

These areas differ in importance, depending on the sport you play and your event or position within it. For example, in golf, the technical and tactical areas are absolutely critical, whereas agility, speed, and endurance play a much lesser role. If you're a sprinter in swimming or track, what's important is to go as fast as possible. Therefore, tactics aren't nearly as important as your technique, agility, and endurance. If you play striker for your soccer team, your strength, agility, speed, flexibility, and endurance are as important as your technical expertise and tactical knowledge of the game.

While there is a constant interplay among these training dimensions, the mental arena provides the glue that holds the other three areas together. Regardless of the sport, what goes on in your head dramatically affects the physical, technical, and tactical performance by either enhancing or diminishing their effectiveness.

Eliminating Causes
of the Slump

Slump busting begins with the athlete or coach examining and then ruling out any physical, technical, or tactical reasons for the consistent bad play. Once you determine that your performance blues don't result from these aspects, you can then move on to the mental arena and Steps 2 through 10 in the slump-busting model. However, should you discover, for example, that your technique is significantly contributing to your poor play, then a change here may be all that you really need to send that slump packing. If that's the case, then Steps 2 through 10 will help you further strengthen your mental toughness and insure that any future problems will be short-lived.

Jose's long-term batting woes demonstrate why it's important to first rule out the nonmental causes of a slump before going after the athlete's mind. A Division I baseball player, Jose has been virtually hitless in well over 30 games. Having always been someone with fairly solid hitting fundamentals, Jose naturally assumed that his slump must be a direct result of his head getting in the way. Certainly his batting problems had done a number on his confidence, not to mention on his aggressiveness at the plate. Recently he noticed that self-doubts were creeping into his fielding.

Because he knew that he was too anxious at the plate, Jose learned some breathing techniques to help calm himself down. He used mental rehearsal, imagining himself at the plate feeling confident and making good contact. He started to work on eliminating the negative self-talk that seemed to accompany his every trip to the plate. But regardless of all his efforts in the mental arena, Jose's hitting continued to slump, until one day his coach noticed something very interesting during batting practice: Jose was ever so slightly mistiming the rotation of his hips on every swing. The coach then briefly worked with Jose to correct this technical problem. In his very next game he went 3 for 4, hitting the ball hard each time.

This one very small but significant mechanical mistake had scuttled Jose's hitting, dragging his confidence down with it. The coach worked with him for no more than 10 minutes and—like magic—Jose's hitting returned to normal. End of slump! Almost immediately his confidence and aggressiveness at the plate returned. There was absolutely nothing wrong with this batter's head that solid technique couldn't correct.

Fortunately, the low confidence caused by his slump did not get in Jose's way once the correct technique was introduced. This is not always the case. Sometimes a slump caused by a physical, technical, or tactical mistake goes on so long that even after it's corrected, low self-confidence takes over to maintain the performance problem. In these situations the athlete or team will significantly benefit from Steps 2 through 10 of the slump-busting model. You must ask yourself this tricky question: Are you stuck in a slump because of your head, or is your mental game completely out of whack because you're stuck in a slump? Only after you've gone through Step 1 in the model can you really begin to answer this question in a useful way.

Tanika, a Division I collegiate distance runner, contacted me after back-to-back disappointing cross-country and winter track seasons. Her times as a sophomore were much slower than the previous year, and her frustrations were getting the best of her. She claimed that she was losing the joy of running, that she frequently cried after practice, and that she was contemplating quitting because of her slump.

When Tanika was a freshman, her coach told her that although she wasn't good enough to qualify for scholarship money, she was certainly welcome to try out for the team. Although Tanika was a little insulted by the coach's frankness, she was determined to prove him wrong. That year she worked harder than she ever had and was a huge asset to the team. She out-trained and out-competed scholarship athletes and was a big point winner at conference championships. The coach relied on her to be a positive, influential team leader. He was clearly pleased with her tremendous efforts and improvements and was delighted to hear that she would be staying around campus over the summer to continue her training. He made a commitment to help her out on a daily basis.

That summer Tanika was excited to begin and wasn't even upset when the coach never showed up for their first scheduled meeting. He apologized that night and agreed to meet with her the next day. When he failed to show up again, she trained with the men's team. For the next three weeks the coach continued to miss every one of their scheduled sessions, so Tanika continued to train alone or with the men. Each time he failed to show, the coach called with his apologies and excuses. Tanika's enthusiasm and motivation slowly began to wane, and in the middle of the summer she decided to take a vacation from training.

At the beginning of her sophomore year Tanika learned that the coach had increased the scholarship money of several of her slower, less committed teammates. In addition, he had recruited and given a full scholarship to another miler for the winter track team who not only was quite a bit slower that Tanika but dropped out of school

→

within the first month of cross-country workouts. While Tanika continued to train consistently, she began to feel more and more resentful toward her coach. She felt that he took her for granted and didn't respect her training ethic or skills. During meets he would tell her that they needed to work on various parts of her technique, but never followed through in practice. When she directly asked him for help he just told her to "run a few more laps."

Tanika did not realize that her anger and frustration were directly related to the coach. She liked him and didn't want to complain. When she started running slower, he didn't know what to do to help her. Her attitude began to spiral downward along with her confidence. Soon, all her races suffered. She couldn't understand why she was racing so poorly.

Tanika's slump had nothing to do with the kinds of mental issues discussed in the remaining chapters. Her problems were directly linked to the misunderstandings and lack of communication between her and her coach. From her freshman year on, Tanika never once told the coach how she was feeling. Consequently, he never had the opportunity to adjust his behavior to correct the problem. I encouraged Tanika to write *all* her concerns down on paper and then present them to the coach. Her feelings about that relationship were getting in the way of her training and competing. The coach's insensitivity to Tanika's feelings further contributed to this problem.

At the end of her sophomore year Tanika sat down with the coach and "put it all on the table." She explained how she had been feeling and how the coach's behavior had hurt her. After their two-hour meeting, Tanika felt like a weight had been lifted off her shoulders. Her coach was receptive to her and took responsibility for some of his behavior that had contributed to the problem. When she started her junior year, Tanika had a partial scholarship and was named the team captain. She had a great junior year and had rediscovered not only her speed, but also her joy in running.

Not every slump is in your head. As this example clearly illustrates, sometimes coaches' behaviors can have a significant impact on the quality of their athletes' performances.

If you're struggling as an athlete, the smartest thing you can do is to first consult with a coach or someone with the tactical, technical, and physical knowledge of your sport. Have your coach examine your mechanics; look at your flexibility, strength, speed, and conditioning; and assess your use and understanding of strategy. If these elements pass inspection, then you

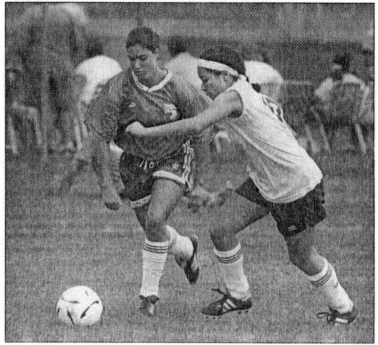

© Mary Langenfeld

can confidently turn to the mental dimension for a solution. Similarly, these areas should be the very first ones that you explore as a coach when you look for answers to your team's slump or an individual's repeated performance woes. Don't automatically assume that you have a mental problem on your hands until you've ruled out these other three performance areas. A slump may clearly look like it's coming from a mental problem, when in actuality something else is going on.

> *If you're struggling as an athlete, the smartest thing you can do is to first consult with a coach or someone with the tactical, technical, and physical knowledge of your sport.*

For example, a high school basketball team started its season by losing seven out of its first nine games. In each loss, the team consistently fell apart toward the end of close games. With seven or eight minutes remaining in regulation time, the players' intensity evaporated, they couldn't make a basket, and they were plagued by turnovers. The only two games that they won were against much weaker opponents. An obvious explanation for the players' predictable collapse was that the team had elevated choking to an art form. Prescription? Bring in a sport "shrink" immediately to help build the players' confidence, improve their focus at crunch time, and teach them how to better handle pressure. Good reasoning, but wrong solution! This team's disappearing act in those tight games was caused by the athletes' bodies, not their minds. As a group they were in terrible physical shape. Shortly after the coach zeroed in on the physical dimension of the game, turning up the heat in practice with intensive endurance training, the team began winning more of its close games.

Another example of a slump caused by physical factors is the case of Jenny, a nine-year-old gymnast who had been immobilized by her fear of a back walkover on the beam for well over six months. Whenever she was asked to attempt this skill, Jenny felt sure she would miss with her hands and hit her head on the beam. She became frozen with fright and unable to move.

No matter what I tried with her mentally, I couldn't neutralize her fear until her coaches and I discovered what should have been obvious: Jenny lacked the physical flexibility to bend over backward and execute this trick successfully. This is why she was afraid! This discovery made solving the problem a whole lot easier. Jenny was given exercises to increase her flexibility, and within two months she had successfully mastered the back walkover.

Testing Your Performance Awareness

So how do you determine the real culprit in your slump? Is it a physical, technical, or tactical factor? Or is it really your head that's wreaking all this havoc? Use the following questionnaire to help you answer this important question. Its purpose is to raise your awareness about your performance so that you can then make the needed changes to bust that slump. Keep in mind that awareness is the first step in change. Before you can fix any problem, you must become familiar with it.

For best results, first answer the questions by yourself. Next, ask your coach or someone else who knows your strengths and weaknesses to answer the questions. It is absolutely critical that you get input from someone besides yourself. Your own awareness is always limited.

To help you further determine whether your slump is being fed by some nonmental factor, get a coach or teammate to videotape your performance. Watching yourself on tape will help you see things that you might ordinarily miss. Perhaps you even have a video recording of a preslump performance. Comparing past and present performances can also help you identify what might be fueling the slump.

PHYSICAL, TECHNICAL, AND TACTICAL QUESTIONNAIRE

■ Physical

Is your slump caused by any of the following?

	What you would say	What your coach would say
Lack of sleep		
Lack of upper-body strength		
Lack of lower-body strength		
Limited agility		
Limited flexibility		
Poor endurance		
Slow foot speed		
Preslump injury		
Preslump sickness		
Inadequate diet		

■ Technical

1. Do you remember changing any aspect of your technique (for example, grip, stance, swing, stroke, or follow-through) before the slump started?
2. Have you deliberately changed any aspect of your technique since the slump began?
3. Do you lack any specific skills that may be directly contributing to your performance difficulties?
4. Have you moved up into a higher competitive level recently?
5. What would your coach say about your technique and mechanics?

■ Tactical

1. Did you change any of your tactics before the slump started? (For example, a tennis player may decide to play more aggressively and attack the net instead of staying in the backcourt; a batter may decide to start pulling the ball more or go after the big hit every time up.)

→

2. Have you changed your tactics since the slump began?

3. Have your tactics remained solid despite your bad play?

4. What would your coach say about your tactical grasp of the sport?

Are You Burned Out?

In ruling out the physical causes of performance problems, you need to consider one additional area. Slumps can be a direct result of overtraining and burnout. If an athlete has been working too hard for too long without adequate rest, then performance will suffer. Chronic fatigue may set in, overuse injuries begin to surface, and performance gets stale. The athlete goes to practice or competitions hoping to just get through and counting the hours and minutes until it's over. This is a TGIF (Thank goodness it's Friday) or burnout mentality. Peak performers, on the other hand, are filled with excitement and anticipation about training. They can't wait to get started. These players are operating from a TGIM (Thank goodness it's Monday) mind-set.

Slumps can be a direct result of overtraining and burnout.

Rest is an important yet frequently overlooked part of training in every sport. Athletes, distracted by a "more is better" philosophy of training, fail to adequately listen to their bodies. As a result they overtrain and allow their bodies too little recovery time. This flawed training regime results in diminishing returns—the more you put in, the less you get out. If your training or competition schedule does not allow enough time for you to recover, then the results often will be burnout and subpar performances.

This was the situation with Barbara, an LPGA golfer who came to me out of frustration because she couldn't seem to play well when it really counted. She did fine in practice but consistently self-destructed in big-money tournaments. She had been on the tour for several years and had yet to have a really successful season. She felt frustrated and talked about packing it all in. She dreaded tournaments and had an "I can't wait until this is over" attitude as she competed. She couldn't remember when she last enjoyed playing.

When I asked what her training schedule was like and how much time she usually took off, she looked at me as if I were speaking a foreign language. She hadn't taken any serious time away from the game for well over two years. Barbara was totally burned out and needed a vacation. This was the main cause of her consistently poor play. After taking four months off, Barbara came back refreshed and looking forward to playing again. For the first time in two years she actually began to enjoy herself out on the course. Her renewed pleasure was almost immediately reflected in her much-improved play.

How about you? Are your performance problems related to overtraining or burnout? Answer the following burnout questionnaire to determine if this is a factor in your slump.

BURNOUT QUESTIONNAIRE

Answer True or False to the following questions:

1. I am tired all the time.
2. I don't enjoy practice the way I used to.
3. When I practice, I frequently wish I were somewhere else.
4. I dread competing.
5. It has been a long time since I really had fun playing.
6. I continually question why I remain in the sport.
7. I find it hard to keep focused on my goals.
8. I seem to get injured more than ever before.
9. My injuries never seem to heal.
10. My attitude seems to have become worse over the past several months.
11. I resent having to sacrifice so much of my time for the sport.
12. I don't handle the discomfort from hard training as well as I did last year.
13. Sometimes I don't even care that I don't care.
14. I'm more negative than usual about myself and my training.
15. I have trouble concentrating in practice.
16. I put myself down a lot lately.
17. I really resent my coach.
18. I have more trouble getting along with teammates than ever before.

→

19. I feel pressured by others to remain in the sport.
20. I don't seem to bounce back from setbacks and losses like I used to.

■ Scoring the Questionnaire

Each True = 1 point; each False = 0 points. Add up the total number of points. If you scored between 1 and 3 out of a possible 20 points, then you probably don't need to be concerned about burnout. Scores between 4 and 7 indicate that you're starting to "cook" and could use some time off. Scores between 8 and 14 indicate that you are in desperate need of a vacation from training and competition. If you scored 15 or higher, then you are seriously burned out and need to sit down with your coach and have a heart-to-heart discussion about your continued involvement in the sport.

Burnout is no joking matter. If you think that your slump comes from being physically out of gas, take note. You will not snap out of this kind of slump by training harder. On the contrary, working harder will only get you more stuck. Sometimes the fastest way to get to a goal is the slowest. Time off from training might be just what the slump doctor ordered to get your performance back on the fast track.

In 1986, just after his 16th birthday, tennis prodigy Andre Agassi turned pro. He brought to the court amazing speed, otherworldly hand-eye coordination, and perhaps the hardest forehand in the game. These skills and his marketable good looks had product sponsors scrambling to get on the Agassi bandwagon, and almost overnight Andre became an international fixture, hawking cameras, sneakers, and more. The tremendous hype surrounding Agassi was further fueled by his sometimes showboating, rude behavior and his habit of tanking sets in big matches to conserve his energy. He incurred the wrath and disdain of opponents as well as tournament organizers with his cocky, seemingly disrespectful behavior while making one final that year and rising to the rank of number 89 in the world.

In his second year, after losing a first-round match in Washington, D.C., he gave his rackets away and vowed to quit the game. Thus began an eight-year period of inconsistency that seemed to both define and plague Agassi. "I'd have one good year and fall to pieces the next," he said.[1] In 1988 he rose to number 3, then fell to number 7 in

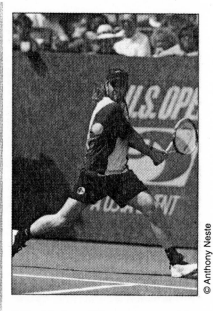

© Anthony Neste

1989. In 1990 Agassi reached the finals of both the French and U.S. Open tournaments and climbed back to number 4. In 1991, he fell back to number 10, losing another French Open final and ending the year on a sour note with a first-round loss in the U.S. Open. After this loss Agassi again considered quitting the game.

To try to turn things around and stop his every-other-year slump, Agassi distanced himself from his hypercritical, demanding father, moving out of his house. Eight months later, in July of 1992, he won Wimbledon. The next year his career took a serious nosedive and nearly crashed for good. In 1993, suffering from a painful wrist injury, he played only 14 tournaments. He gained eight pounds and watched his ranking fall to number 24. At the same time Nick Bolleteri, his coach of 10 years, sent Agassi a letter ending their relationship.

Injured, overweight, out of shape and seemingly in a free fall, Agassi appeared headed for oblivion. Even his brother Phillip was quoted as saying that he doubted Andre would ever be able to come back. Then Brad Gilbert, a veteran tour player, became Agassi's new coach. Gilbert detailed Agassi's weaknesses and taught him that physical talent was only half the secret to success. "I've always had a gift," Agassi said, "and my talent has gotten me through a lot of tough things. But I've never actually understood my responsibility to that talent, which is to go out there and be so focused on what I need to do, dedicate myself, and understand what I need to do to make my talent come through."[2] In March of 1994 Gilbert began to overhaul Agassi's game and attitude. Agassi began working with Gil Reyes, a personal trainer, and soon his body began to take on a new shape. His coach and trainer helped him curb his immense appetite for junk food, and Agassi's once visible belly was replaced by washboard abs. They worked on his physical endurance so that he would get stronger rather than weaker as a tournament progressed. Gilbert got Agassi to creatively

→

think through his points and to plan for his matches instead of thoughtlessly belting the ball.

The results of all these efforts were transforming. By the end of 1994 Agassi had beaten every player in the top 10 during a nine-month surge that lifted him to number 2. That year he won the U.S. Open and seemed to be a serious contender for best in the world. In 1995 Agassi continued to excel, winning the Australian Open and trading the number 1 spot with Pete Sampras for most of the year. Despite limited playing time in 1996 due to an injury, Agassi's new attitude, approach to the game, and physical conditioning snapped his slump and put him back in contention.

Conclusion

After you've been able to clearly rule out physical, tactical, and technical causes, and you're sure that your problems aren't related to burnout, then you're ready to go on to the next step in my slump-busting model. There we will address the mental side of your performance and begin to build mental toughness. First we will work on restoring your feelings of power and control. Most slumping athletes have tried everything in their power to break free from the clutches of the slump. Because they have consistently failed in these attempts, many are left feeling powerless and out of control. Step 2 in slump busting is about understanding that you have the power to turn that slump around and to emerge from your difficulties as a stronger competitor. It will help you move from feelings of helplessness and hopelessness to those of strength and hope.

2

ESTABLISHING SELF-CONTROL

"It's not what's happening around you,
It's not what's happening to you,
What really matters is what's happening inside you."

—Dr. Rob Gilbert

So are you ready to take the next step? You've been able to determine clearly that your problem isn't physical, technical, or tactical. You're in relatively good shape, have decent mechanics, and possess a solid understanding of your sport's strategies, yet you still can't seem to break free from that slump's nasty clutches. While you may be burning up with frustration, you're fairly sure that you're not burned out. A rest is *not* what you need right now! If this description fits you, then it's a good bet that your slump is linked to your head—the final key area of training. To snap out of your performance doldrums, you must now venture into that terrifying and uncharted wilderness between your ears: your mind.

If you're like most athletes and coaches, you're used to being in control of your "athletic destiny." As a serious athlete, you know that with the right amount of hard work, sacrifice, and good coaching, you can accomplish almost anything. Before your performance troubles, you probably felt in control of yourself and your body. You felt a sense of pride and accomplishment from your ability to meet obstacles and defeat them. You were used to being the master of your body, knowing that a strong will could almost always prevail over aching muscles, strained ligaments, and even broken bones to get you closer to your goals. Failures, setbacks, and injuries, while temporarily knocking you off track, only seemed to fuel your determination to succeed.

Tim Daggett, 1984 Olympic gold medal gymnast, demonstrated this tenacious attitude over the course of his remarkable career. Daggett had four "career-ending" injuries as a gymnast but simply refused to give up control and abandon his dream. After one of these injuries, nine different doctors told him that his problem was serious enough to require neck surgery and that, of course, he would never be able to compete again. Undeterred, Daggett found a tenth physician who thought that such an operation was too radical and prescribed traction, rest, and intensive rehabilitation instead. Nine months later, Tim was back in the gym seriously training again!

Your talent doesn't have to be Olympic-caliber for you to relate to this refuse-to-quit mind-set. Many athletes derive motivation from obstacles and setbacks. The tougher things get, the tougher the athlete gets. If you're like this, then feelings of power and control are your constant companions. Sure, you may have the occasional self-doubts and fleeting feelings of inadequacy like the rest of us. But as a committed athlete, you usually feel in control of yourself and powerful. . . *until now!*

The slump nullifies your strongest weapon—your work ethic—and turns it against you. Perhaps when something in your physical game caused a performance problem you had the tenacity and discipline to work through the difficulty, no matter what! However, this dependable strategy is not working now. Trying harder and spending more time not only will not cure the mind-based slump, but actually will make it worse! It's like getting stuck in quicksand and physically struggling to get free. The harder and more desperate your efforts, the faster and deeper you sink. Your attempts to find a solution only contribute to the problem.

> *M*ost attempts at slump busting fail because athletes look outside themselves for the culprit.

This effect is what makes slumps so upsetting. Since they don't seem to be caused by anything physical, mechanical, or strategic in your game (assuming you've ruled out these causes in Step 1), they do not respond to your normal remedies. They don't give you—the athlete who is used to taking charge—anything concrete to attack. It's as if you're in a game where the rules suddenly change, and now your best moves are useless. The strategies that solve a conditioning problem do not work when the cause of the slump is mental. Most attempts at slump busting fail because athletes look outside themselves for the culprit when they should be looking in the mirror for both the problem and the solution.

Stopping the Slide

When continued attempts to bust a slump fail, your confidence is shaken to the core. Self-doubts creep in, and as your self-confidence begins to crack, your familiar feelings of control and effectiveness begin to slip away. A nasty feeling creeps in that any action you take will make no difference. Everything seems to be sliding downhill.

The longer a slump has its claws in you, the more powerless and hopeless you feel. Attacking and erasing these feelings of powerlessness—the second step in the slump-busting model—*is your first important job mentally.* To restore your confidence and energy, you first must recognize that *your loss of control is only an illusion.* That is, despite your performance problems, you are still very much in control. While you may not be using it, you *still* have the power. Understanding that the power and control reside within you is critical to successfully working through the other eight steps in the slump-busting model to end your performance problems and develop mental toughness.

A ttacking and erasing feelings of powerlessness—the second step in the slump-busting model—is your first important job mentally.

Knowing that you already have the key to unlock the slump will enable you to take control of your focus (Step 3), confront your fears (Step 4), change your beliefs to expect success (Step 5), develop performance-enhancing imagery (Step 6), set slump-busting and peak-performance goals (Step 7), build self-confidence (Step 8), master failures and setbacks (Step 9), and avoid future slumps (Step 10).

How do you convince yourself that you have the control to turn the slump around when overwhelming evidence to the contrary is piling up all around you? Yes, you may have elevated choking to an art form. Sure, your slump may have plagued you for months. Of course you're frustrated, but before you pack it in you need to understand that there is actually a good reason why you haven't been performing well! Contrary to popular myths, your slump is *not* an airborne, invisible virus that mysteriously attacks its unsuspecting athlete-host. A slump is mostly logical and understandable if you examine its development and your own role in maintaining it.

As you're probably painfully aware, athletic performance is not always consistent. You won't be at your best *all* the time. The road of your sports career winds up and down through peaks and valleys and is littered with potholes all along the way. These off times are a *natural* and expected part of sports, even for the very best athletes. You go out to play and discover that no matter what you do, your performance is just plain flat. Your fastball doesn't have any zip. You have no feel for the water. You seem to have left your jump shot in the locker room. Your tennis racket feels like a dead fish. You sprain an ankle or strain ligaments, or perhaps you fall off the beam or hit your head on the diving board. These physical and emotional bumps and bruises are a *normal* part of competition. *Keeping this perspective is critical to getting yourself back in control.*

Most athletes do not realize that these tough times create a perfect climate for a slump to grow and flourish. The majority of mental-based slumps get their start during performance valleys because these bad performances, heartbreaking losses, or injuries actually are the *seeds* of a slump. While they don't cause the slump directly, they create the slump's opportunity.

For example, failing to hit safely four games in a row is frustrating, but this string of empty at-bats doesn't cause your slump or even mean that you're in a slump. Getting lost in the middle of a dive and hitting your head on the board may be painful, but by itself doesn't directly lead to a performance block. Missing two clutch free throws that cost your team the game doesn't mean that from now on you'll choke at crunch time. Whether these events have any lasting power over you and develop into a slump directly depends on *what you say to yourself about them and how you view them*. Like a seed, these events cannot take root and grow out of control unless you get out the shovel and watering can and plant them.

> **W**hether events have any lasting power over you and develop into a slump directly depends on what you say to yourself about them and how you view them.

The batter plants the seeds of a slump by *remembering* how many times he hasn't hit as he's loosening up on deck. He may question himself as he steps into the batter's box: "What if I don't get a hit? What if I strike out *again*? What if coach benches me?" The diver does this kind of "mental planting" when she takes a trip down memory lane the next time she has to perform the same dive on which she originally got hurt. Because of the fear and anxiety that she dredged up from the past, she worries that the mistake might happen again. The same anxieties can cripple the basketball player. Perhaps he keeps reminding himself that he's a "choke artist." Then when he steps to the line the next time the pressure is on, his thoughts will be on failure and his shooting will reflect this.

Because these preperformance thoughts and self-talk tighten muscles, choke off breathing, erode confidence, and distract the athletes from a winning focus, the athletes unknowingly set themselves up to fail again and again. Slumps, therefore, can only take root and flourish if *you* give them enough negative airtime in your mind. If you are struggling with a slump, then you are doing things in your head *right now* that are keeping your performance woes alive and well. This is the good news, because it means that if you change your mental strategies, you can get yourself unstuck and back in control!

Determining Your Mental Strategies

To understand your slump and your role in it, identify what you are doing in your mind just before and during the performance—what you are thinking, focusing on, "seeing," and saying to yourself. Poor mechanics or tactics would quickly send your performance down the tubes; so too would poor mental mechanics or strategies. *To bust that slump, you must first recognize your slump-feeding mental strategies and replace them with performance-enhancing ones.* To help you identify your present counterproductive mental strategies, complete the following exercise.

WHAT MENTAL STRATEGIES ARE YOU USING?

■ Part 1

Pick two or three examples of past performances that clearly represent your slump. For example: In your last dual meet, you once again choked in the final 25 meters of the race. You got up to do a back sommie on the beam and balked *again!* You threw an interception when the game was on the line. You lost again to that same opponent. You let a weaker player continually beat you to the ball.

Taking each performance separately, answer the following questions *in as much detail as possible* and record your responses:

1. What were your *thoughts and self-talk* in the days leading up to and the day of the performance?
2. What *imagery* was in your mind before the performance?
3. What was the nature of your self-talk and thoughts *right before* the performance?
4. Did you have any *preperformance expectations?* If so, what were they?
5. What thoughts and self-talk did you have *during* the performance?
6. When you made mistakes, what did you *think and say* to yourself?
7. What were your thoughts and self-talk *after* the performance?

→

Answer Questions 1 through 7 for each specific example of the slump. Compare your answers for each experience. Do you notice a common theme in your responses? Was your self-talk similar before each performance? Was your concentration focused on negative outcomes in each performance? Your thoughts, self-talk, focus, imagery, and expectations are your mental strategies for a performance. If your mental strategies are negative and self-defeating, they will keep you stuck in your slump!

■ Part 2

Pick two or three examples from peak performances when you were not struggling with a slump. You can include examples from parts of your game that are presently unaffected by the slump (for example, you're in a hitting slump but your fielding is still fine), or you can think back to preslump performances. Answer Questions 1 through 7 for each of these positive experiences. Look for a common mental theme in these responses. What was your self-talk before and during these performances? Did you notice a consistent focus? How did you deal with miscues during these performances? Your thoughts, self-talk, focus, imagery, and expectations during your peak performances are positive mental strategies that enhance performance—*strategies you can use again to bust that slump!*

■ Part 3

Compare the mental strategies you identified in Parts 1 and 2. What *specific* differences do you see in your preperformance self-talk and focus of concentration? Do you think and talk to yourself more when you are slumping? When the going gets rough during both good and bad performances, how do you handle the setbacks in each case? What do you concentrate on during a slumping performance as compared with a great one?

While the results of the comparison in this exercise may be obvious, the implications are very important. First, there is nothing random about your slump. It is directly related to your *unknowing* use of bad mental strategies. Many people think that the slump *causes* the negativity, faulty focus, and expectations of failure. This conclusion is actually backward. While everyone goes through down times in their performances, what *you* do *mentally* with those down times is critical. The real culprit here is your mental strategies. Your negativity, misdirected concentration, and self-doubts cause the slump.

As shown in the following list, there is a clear difference between the mental strategies of a slump and those of a peak performance. The heartache and frustration that struggling athletes experience can be directly connected to their thoughts, self-talk, imagery, and focus of concentration, before and during performances. These strategies are markedly different when athletes are at the top of their game from when they are not. How do your answers from the previous exercise compare with the mental strategies listed? Can you see some clear mental differences between your best and worst performances? Your *awareness* of the differing mental strategies in good and bad performances forms the basis from which you can bust that slump and take back control.

Armed with this awareness, you can use the techniques presented in *Sports Slump Busting* to develop more positive mental strategies and get yourself back in control. For example, once you know that your performance focus is faulty, Step 3 in the model ("Developing a Championship Focus") will teach you how to concentrate correctly. If your self-talk is negative and

THE MENTAL STRATEGIES OF PEAK AND SLUMPING PERFORMANCE

Mental Strategies	Slumping Performance	Peak Performance
Thoughts	Negative, self-depreciating	Positive, supportive
Self-talk	Confidence-eroding	Confidence-enhancing
Focus	On uncontrollables or outcomes	On controllables or on the process rather than the outcome
Imagery	"See" what you're afraid will happen	"See" what you want to happen

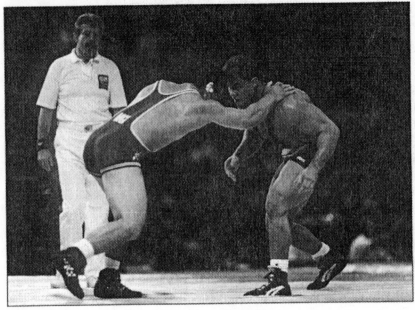

© Claus Andersen

confidence-eroding, Steps 5 and 8 ("Expecting Success" and "Building Self-Confidence") will teach you how to turn this "inner coaching" around and believe in yourself again. If you're aware that your internal images are negative and performance-disrupting, Step 6 ("Developing Positive Images") will help you replace them with more performance-enhancing "movies."

As you proceed through each step of the model, be sure to refer to your answers in the exercise on pages 27-28 (especially those in Part 1 regarding bad performances) to see if that step's slump-busting strategies directly address one of your weaknesses.

Getting Back in Control

Starting *right now* you can begin to take back control. You can learn to change those slump-feeding mental strategies. Many of the thoughts that bounce around inside your skull give power and control to people and circumstances outside you. Getting back in control depends on your awareness of these thoughts and how much power you are unknowingly giving away. An important question to ask yourself here is, "How much am I participating in keeping myself stuck?" To find the answer, take the following short test.

WHO'S IN CONTROL?

Answer T if the statement is generally true for you or F if the statement is generally false.

1. I worry about my opponent's size, strength, or speed before I compete.

2. The temperature during the competition can negatively affect me.

3. When the conditions of the competition site are terrible, I tend to lose my confidence.

4. Faulty equipment or apparatus distracts me and hinders my performance.

5. Opponents who cheat have virtually no impact on me.

6. I perform better when few people watch.

7. I tend to dwell on mistakes by the officials.

8. Overly aggressive opponents often take me out of my game.

9. A screaming, heckling crowd amuses me and I can easily forget about them.

10. I spend too much time wondering what the coaches think of me.

11. My coaches just seem to add to my performance troubles.

12. It bothers me when opponents talk trash or try to psych me out.

13. My parents can have a big impact on how I perform.

14. I don't think my coach really believes in me.

15. I love being the underdog.

16. It doesn't take much to psych me out.

17. My parents' (or others') expectations get in my way.

18. If I had better coaching, I wouldn't be in a slump.

19. If my pregame rituals get upset, so does my performance.

20. I can't perform well if I feel like I haven't had a good warm-up.

21. When I do well, I feel it was just luck.

22. I don't really care about my opponent's record or reputation.

23. I sometimes feel that I'll never get over my slump.

24. The unexpected rarely knocks me off track.

25. My teammates add to my performance blues.

→

■ Scoring

T = 1, F = 0 for Questions 1–4, 6–8, 10–14, 16–21, 23, and 25
T = 0, F = 1 for Questions 5, 9, 15, 22, and 24

■ Interpreting Your Score

There are 25 possible points on this test. The higher your score, the less in control you feel and the more power you attribute to outside factors or people. The closer your score is to zero, the more in control of yourself you feel. High scores (15 and up) indicate that you are feeding your slump with mental strategies that overfocus on factors outside your control. Simply put, you see yourself as a rowboat in a storm, being tossed every which way and going nowhere. Scores from 6 to 14 similarly reflect a control problem, but at least you occasionally use your oars to try to set a course. If you scored between 0 and 5, then you feel in control most of the time, like the captain of your ship.

If you're slumping or stuck and your scores indicate a lack of control, try not to worry. The strategies in *Sports Slump Busting* will systematically help you get back in control and smooth sailing will soon follow. Starting with the next section, you'll learn to recognize the biggest cause of slumps and low confidence.

Mastering the Uncontrollables

When you as an athlete focus on the uncontrollables at any point *before* or *during* performance, several things happen. First, your stress goes up—your breathing speeds up and your muscles tighten. Second, your confidence falls. Third, as a result of the first two effects, your performance goes down the proverbial tubes.

The uncontrollables are all those things that you have no *direct* control over when you perform, but that most athletes invariably complain about: the officiating; the field and playing conditions; the weather; the time of day that you have to compete; the skill level, size, strength, and style of play of your opponents; your teammates; your coaches; the fans; parents' or other people's expectations; anything negative in the past, like a mistake, a previous failure, or an injury; and anything negative that might happen in the future, like losing or messing up.

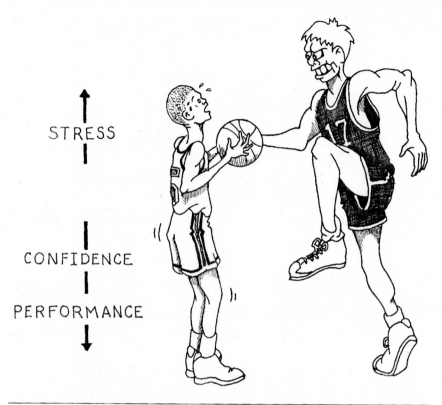

STRESS

CONFIDENCE

PERFORMANCE

The slump and the uncontrollables.

One of the principles of peak performance discussed in the introduction is maintaining a "process focus." By concentrating on what you are doing while you are doing it and not jumping ahead to the outcome, you can maximize your chances of performing to your potential. Many performance-disrupting uncontrollables (for example, winning or losing, getting or not getting a hit, and so on) are related to the outcome and therefore violate this important principle.

As a general rule, a focus on uncontrollables will almost always set an athlete or team up for repeated failure. Such a focus seriously erodes your feelings of personal power and causes choking and intimidation. The slump and uncontrollables go hand-in-hand. Your ability to overcome fears (Step 4), develop confidence (Steps 5 and 8), master failure (Step 9), and effectively handle the pressure of performance and avoid future slumps (Step 10) is directly related to your focus on performance uncontrollables.

For example, I recently worked with Southern Connecticut State University's (SCSU) men's soccer team before its Division II quarterfinal game of the NCAA Championship. They had to play *away* against an equally

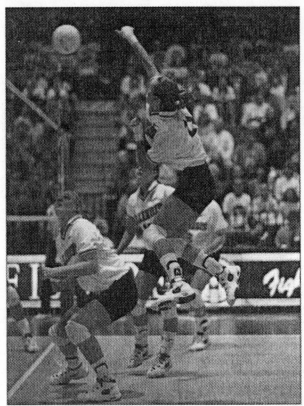

© Daily Illini

talented team that *played extremely aggressively* and was tough to beat at home. In *last year's quarterfinal loss* on the same field, the SCSU Owls dropped a game that, according to their coach, they should have won. The Owls got distracted by the *lousy field conditions*, the *extremely wet and cold weather*, *inconsistent officiating*, *fans who they felt were abusive and totally out of control*, and the *overly aggressive play of their opponents*. A focus on all these uncontrollables (in italics) caused the Owls to fall apart.

A few of the returning SCSU players remembered this loss and were using it to fuel their intensity. The majority of the athletes, however, were negatively focusing on the uncontrollables as the game approached. Had their team gone into the game with this faulty focus, they very well may have lost again. In turn, this second loss may have formed the basis of a minislump ("Whenever we play this team, we lose."). Instead, I reminded the Southern players of what they already knew: "Focus on the uncontrollables and you'll self-destruct. Every time you're confronted by an uncontrollable, recognize it for what it is and quickly bring your focus of concentration back to the game and what you can control."

In this year's quarterfinal game, SCSU was confronted with many uncontrollables (in italics below) that easily could have diverted their concentration. Not only were they playing in front of a *hostile crowd*, but the game had to be *postponed* because of a *snow-covered field*. The Owls *didn't even get a chance to practice for two days*. Southern had also *lost its last game of the year here a month and a half before*, when their opponents scored two goals in the last 2:49. The Owls had to play almost half the game, including two overtime periods and a sudden death, *one man down (a Southern player was red-carded during regulation)*! On top of all this, Southern had to *come from behind twice* to win in sudden death.

E*very time you're confronted by an uncontrollable, recognize it and quickly bring your focus of concentration back to what you can control.*

Whether we're talking about a team's play or your individual efforts, a focus on the uncontrollables will almost always knock you off track and trash your performance. I say "almost always" here because there are a few athletes who consistently play better when they focus on their opponents' size, skill, or reputation, or on the fans' hostility. If you are this kind of athlete, keep doing what works for you. The general rule doesn't apply to you for these uncontrollables. However, you must be alert to a focus on the other uncontrollables, which can undermine your performance.

While so many things are uncontrollable, the one thing that you can learn to control is your reaction. If you're presently struggling with a slump, controlling your reaction may seem virtually impossible to you. But keep in mind that you may be feeling so out of control mainly because of your mental strategy of zooming in on the uncontrollables before and during performance. Uncontrollables will continue to be part of the scenery of competitive sports. Reestablishing your control is about spotting them right away and then deliberately steering clear of them by refocusing your attention on the things you *can* control.

Imagine you're riding a bicycle down a winding path. The path is littered with massive potholes (the uncontrollables) big enough to swallow you, bicycle and all. What do you have to do to insure that you don't end up at the bottom of one of these holes?

Simple! You have to keep yourself focused on the road, so that you can see those holes early enough to navigate around them. If you don't see them, you'll end up in them. This is the case with any uncontrollable, whether it's an opposing quarterback throwing touchdowns or a fan hurling wisecracks. You have to first know what uncontrollables "push your

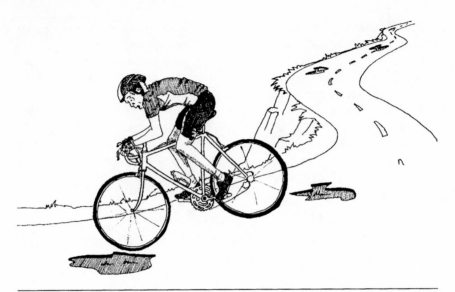

Steering clear of the uncontrollables.

buttons" so you can avoid them by refocusing on something more controllable before or during the performance.

Take a moment right now to think about your slump. Are you inadvertently feeding it by focusing on uncontrollables? If so, what specific uncontrollables haunt you? Write these down. Get to know them. Do you conjure up past failures before you perform? Do visions of possible mistakes dance in your head? Are you overly concerned about your opponent's build and game stats? Do mistakes or bad breaks stick to you like glue? You will begin to regain your power and self-confidence as an athlete when you take control of the concentration piece of your mental strategies.

Using the Uncontrollables as Your Competitive Edge

But why just be content with regaining control? How about using your knowledge of the uncontrollables not only to strengthen your mental toughness, but also to develop a competitive edge over your competition?

When you're performing well, the uncontrollables that pop up during performances are totally irrelevant. They simply have no effect on you. Uncontrollables only have power when things aren't going well or you're stressed to the max. When I was at my best on the tennis court, nothing ever seemed to bother me. The wind, temperature, court conditions, crowd, bad calls, and even my own stupid mistakes all seemed to just bounce off me. However, when I struggled, I'd turn into a detective and go looking for things that could upset me, like the color of my opponent's shirt, the sound of the grass growing, or wind gusts of up to 1 mph. In these situations, uncontrollables are like magnets in their power to pull you or anyone else off center. By anticipating the impact of the uncontrollables on your competition, you can use them as a confidence booster.

When we were first introduced, Tony was a high school junior wrestler who described himself as a "head case." He was an intense competitor who trained diligently but just couldn't seem to win the big matches. He would go 33 matches in a row without a loss during the season and then fall apart in the state tournament. Whenever he competed in an important tournament, his skills, strategy, and instincts would mysteriously vanish and he'd suddenly find himself attempting moves against his opponent that he knew were wrong or useless for the situation he was in. In less important competitions he'd usually win easily by wrestling brilliantly. During his sophomore year Tony qualified for state and lost in the first round. Junior year he won district and sectional and was seeded third in state when he again lost in the first round to someone he had previously beaten easily. His Jekyll and Hyde routine had been going on since freshman year, and now that his junior season was over he had only one more shot at his big goal before college: to win state.

Tony was completely baffled as to what was actually going on. He couldn't understand why he always seemed to lose when it counted the most, especially since he wasn't overly nervous or intimidated going into these bigger matches. As we began to explore his pre- and during-match mental strategies, Tony inadvertently highlighted the real cause of his performance slump. It seemed that before all his good matches Tony followed a strict routine of separating himself from the team and going through a series of stretches and practice moves, all while he was pacing back and forth. As he went through his shadow drills, set-ups, and fakes he would think about what he was going to do to "destroy" his opponent. His self-talk centered around how ready he was physically and mentally and his attention was completely focused on exactly what he was going to do during the match. Furthermore, he was very aware that once the match started his thinking stopped and his instincts took over. After many of these matches he'd be unable to remember the details of what had just happened other than the fact that he had wrestled well.

All of the big matches that Tony had lost were against weaker opponents. In *every* one of these matches Tony did *not* go through his

→

prematch ritual and his mental strategies had almost nothing to do with the match he was about to engage in. Instead he would think things like, "This won't be much of a match, who's next?" or "I killed him last time, what's for dinner?" After these preliminary thoughts he did not talk to himself about his readiness, nor did he focus on his match strategy. When the match started, instead of being in an automatic, nonthinking state, Tony would find his mind racing, especially after he fell behind. Thoughts like, "I gotta make up for this deficit," "I'm wrestling stupidly," and "What's wrong with me?" would plague him throughout the match and further interfere with his performance.

The crucial difference between Tony's good and bad matches was in his mental strategies, self-talk, and focus. Tony had never stopped to closely examine how they related to his disappointing losses. He had been completely unaware that he was changing his mental strategies when he got into the bigger matches. His developing awareness of this difference became a catalyst that helped him very quickly end his slump and get back in control. The summer before his senior year, he wrestled in two prestigious tournaments. Being seeded number 1 in the first tournament, he made sure that during his early-round matches he strictly adhered to the pre-match ritual and self-talk that always accompanied his great matches. As a result, he breezed through the tournament to win, surprising even himself at how well he wrestled. In the second tournament he lost in the final, but was again able to stay on top of his mental strategies early and wrestled well throughout.

Tony's senior year was a continuation of the success of the summer. He lost only once during the regular season, won both district and sectional, and qualified for a second seed in the state tournament. In his first- and second-round matches he easily dominated his opponents with a confident, powerful style of wrestling. He made sure before these matches that his thoughts were locked on his match and that his self-talk generated confidence and intensity. He continued to wrestle well right through to the finals. In the championship match against the number 1 seed he wrestled the match of his life only to lose by one point at the last second. Although he fell short of his goal, he walked off the mat feeling like a champion, happy that he had ended his high school career on an up note.

For example, in most outdoor sports, the weather can have a dramatic impact on field and playing conditions. As a massive uncontrollable, the weather frequently drives athletes up the wall. Windy conditions make it almost impossible for a tennis player to establish good position and timing. Hitting into the wind is no picnic for the ballplayer and gives the pitcher a tremendous advantage. Extreme cold and snow make it tough to get your footing on the football or soccer field and interfere with smooth execution. Excessive heat and humidity quickly drain your strength and endurance, slowing you down on the track. Rain turns playing fields into slippery bogs, interfering with your ability to perform to your potential.

> ***B****y anticipating the impact of the uncontrollables on your competition, you can use them as a confidence booster.*

When stressed by these uncontrollable weather extremes, many athletes lose their game focus and confidence. *You* don't have to! Get into the habit of thinking of the weather or any other uncontrollable as your secret advantage. *You* know that weather and playing conditions are uncontrollable. *You* know that if you focus on them, you'll stress yourself out. *You* know that under this stress, almost everyone else will focus on the uncontrollable, perhaps looking for an excuse to hang their frustrations and mistakes on. Since *you can control* your concentration and response to the uncontrollables, you can use this knowledge as a confidence booster. You don't have to get excited about the lousy weather. You can even hate it! Just don't focus on it! Leave that bad habit for your opponents.

When the Uncontrollables Are People

As we conclude this step, I want to address one additional issue that contributes to the slumping athlete's feelings of powerlessness: the impact of other people on performance. Can your slump be caused by someone else? Do your coaches, parents, teammates, fans, or the media have the power to send you to the performance outhouse?

Certainly coaches occasionally say and do incredibly annoying things that directly assault your confidence. Maybe before the big competition the coach said something unhelpful or even insulting. Perhaps the coach assigned you a role on the team that reduced your playing time. You were in the starting lineup early in the season, but when you began to struggle, the coach benched you! Certainly this new role on the pine and what you see as a vote of no confidence from the coach can fuel your slump. But can the coach or anyone else actually *cause* the slump?

The people around you—coaches, parents, fans, and reporters—can indeed have a significant impact on your performance. How they treat you and what they say about you can, if you take it to heart, undermine your belief in yourself and contribute to your performance problems.

For example, a Division I running back entered his senior year having rushed for over 1,000 yards in the previous two seasons. For some unknown reason, his running game went into a tailspin and after almost three-quarters of the season, he had accumulated barely 300 yards. His coaches couldn't understand what was wrong and frequently lost patience with him. His father was overly critical and wouldn't stop highlighting his son's mistakes. But these assaults to his confidence paled in comparison to how the sportswriters handled his troubles. The local sports media wasted no time in cruelly labeling him as "overrated," a "flash-in-the-pan," and a "dud." Each week they overanalyzed everything he did, looking for yet another failing. It was no wonder that both before and during every game, this player was obsessed with what "they" were going to say about him next. Who's to blame for his slump? Coaches? Father? Sportswriters?

From our discussion of the uncontrollables you know the answer to this question. Everyone except you is an uncontrollable. The actions, comments, and expectations of those around you are usually out of your control. Can they cause your slump? No! Can they make things miserable for

How to Handle Coaches, Parents, the Media, and Fans

- Don't waste your time and energy blaming others, even if you're right.
- Focus on what you *can* control, not what you *can't*.
- Ask coaches what you can do to turn things around.
- If your coaches are saying or doing something unhelpful, give them clear, respectful feedback on the impact of their behavior.
- If a coach is negative and unresponsive, find another coach who listens and can help you keep your perspective in dealing with the first coach.
- If your parents are saying upsetting things, *be direct* in telling them that their comments are not helpful. Then tell them exactly what you need them to say or do to be supportive.
- If your parents cannot be constructive, ask your coach for help.
- Remember to keep *your* goals in mind, not anyone else's.
- Don't allow yourself to get carried away with either positive or negative attention from the fans or media.

you? Absolutely! Can they kill your confidence? Definitely! Can they fuel your slump? No question! But they can't destroy your performance without your permission. Their power over you comes directly from the power you give them.

Billy, a collegiate baseball player, slipped into a batting slump midway through his junior year and, for the first time ever, was benched by his coach. Because he had dreams of someday making it to the majors, Billy worried that his lack of playing time would reduce his chances of being seen by a pro scout. Unfortunately for Billy, his coach was neither communicative nor supportive. When Billy did get an at-bat, his overconcern with getting a hit and frustration with the coach caused him to press. Pressing only contributed to his batting slump and led to even more time on the bench. Billy blamed the coach for his low self-confidence and the slump. Not until this ballplayer switched his concentration from the coach to what he could control was he able to reverse his downward performance spiral.

While maintaining your confidence after being benched by the coach or trashed by the media is difficult, it is not impossible. Blaming others for your extended performance troubles is like blaming a referee for losing the big game. Referees, like coaches, parents, and the media, make bad calls from time to time. So your complaints may even be justified. However, you have to ask yourself an important question: Would you rather be right or bust out of that slump into peak performance? As a huge uncontrollable, coaches, referees, parents, and reporters don't cause you to self-destruct. You have to take the credit for that one! To get back in control, you need to keep focused on yourself and no one else.

> ***T**o get back in control, you need to keep focused on yourself and no one else.*

· However, a coach or parent can help you break the slump. Dave is a classic case in point. In the beginning of the season, before his slump, he was batting .380 as the leadoff hitter. Then his hitting went into the dumpster, dropping his average to .220. Feeling totally worthless, he asked the coach before a game to take him out of the leadoff position because he "really wasn't getting it done for the team." The coach looked him straight in the eye and said, "Son, you were my leadoff hitter when our season started, and you're going to be my leadoff hitter when the season ends. Now get outta here. We've got a game to play." Dave left the coach's office but forgot to take his slump with him. He went 3 for 4 that game and continued to hit consistently the rest of the season.

Certainly the coach's vote of confidence helped Dave start hitting again, in the same way that Billy's coach inadvertently contributed to prolonging

COACHING TIPS FOR SLUMPING ATHLETES

Don'ts

- Don't remind the athletes how long they have been performing badly.
- Don't compare the athletes' past great performances with their present poor ones (unless you're using the past ones as a constructive model for the present).
- Don't disparage the athletes with labels like "stupid," "head case," or "choker."
- Don't penalize the athletes because they are performing badly.
- Don't give the athletes the silent treatment or ignore them.
- Don't be negative.
- Don't focus the athletes' attention on everything they're doing wrong. Instead, help them focus on what they need to do right to improve.

Dos

- Do be empathetic. Step inside their shoes and let them know you understand how it feels to struggle.
- Do be supportive. Build the athletes' confidence and self-esteem. The last thing slumping athletes need is to have others put them down.
- Do communicate clearly, directly, and often. Let the athletes know where they stand, how you feel about their struggle, and what they can do to get through it. If you bench them, help them understand why you're doing it and what they need to do to get back in the game.
- Do be positive and hopeful. Help them believe that their performance problems are only temporary and that they'll get through them.
- Do help them deal constructively with negative actions from parents, fans, and the media. Help them maintain proper perspective when dealing with other people.

his slump by limiting his playing time. Unfortunately, as an athlete you cannot dictate how those around you will act or what circumstances you'll have to face. Thus, all the responsibility for slump busting is on your shoulders, where it belongs.

Conclusion

While your performance problems may have left you feeling helpless, you don't have to remain that way. Your first major step in regaining your power and busting that slump lies with the understanding that you're *still* in control. Slumps get their start from *your* thinking, self-talk, focus, and expectations (mental strategies). This is the good news, because they can't grow out of control if *you* stop using slump-nurturing mental strategies. By first recognizing these inner strategies and your role in maintaining your performance difficulties, you can begin to systematically break the slump cycle and get back in control.

In the next step, "Developing a Championship Focus," you will learn how to block out the uncontrollables and develop slump-busting concentration. Since your performance-related concentration is one of the keys to athletic excellence, this step will help you take another major leap toward restoring your confidence, reestablishing control, and developing mental toughness.

3

DEVELOPING A CHAMPIONSHIP FOCUS

"Yesterday is a canceled check. Tomorrow is a promissory note. Today is the only cash that you have. Spend it wisely."

In any athletic performance, concentration is an important key to excellence. When you're ready physically and have the necessary experience in the sport, the outcome of your training rests almost completely on *how* and *where* you concentrate. Your concentration synthesizes all your training efforts into a laser-like point of energy that burns through obstacles and distractions to accurately zero in on the challenge of the moment. However, when it's misdirected or diffused, your competitive focus can weaken you, undercutting and neutralizing even the best of training regimes.

As you learned in Step 2, focusing on uncontrollables raises anxiety, lowers confidence, and sabotages performance. Therefore, faulty focus of concentration is a major culprit in causing and maintaining a slump. By learning to consistently control what you concentrate on, you can break the slump, restore your confidence, and unlock your peak performance. In Step 2, you learned to recognize your mental strategies—the thoughts, self-talk, and focus that you tend to use before and during a performance. You also learned the role that negative mental strategies play in causing and maintaining your slump. Now, in Step 3, you will learn how to redirect one of your mental strategies—your focus of concentration—to promote peak performance rather than feed a slump.

A *faulty focus of concentration is a major culprit in causing and maintaining a slump.*

An athlete's or team's *focus of concentration* is an essential element in peak and slumping performance. Your focus both before and during performance determines how well you'll handle pressure and influences the consistency and quality of your performance. A misdirected focus underlies almost all slumps.

You can have two different general points of concentration when you practice and compete. One will enhance your performance; the other will undermine it. When your concentration is locked in the experience of what you're doing, you will most likely perform to your physical abilities. When you slip into "the zone," you are totally absorbed in *what* you're doing, *while* you're doing it, without thinking or analyzing.

For example, a swimmer in the midst of peak performance may focus on the feel of the water, the feel of her arm extension on each stroke, the roll of her hips, or the approach of the wall in front of her, all important cues that enable the swimmer to go fast. Similarly, a defensive lineman can react with explosive speed while keeping focused on his blocking assignment and the play as it develops around him.

When you're "on" as an athlete, this "in-the-experience" focus locks you onto the instantaneously developing cues within the performance that enable you to respond with perfect feel, touch, strength, and timing. You pick up the pitcher's release point early and can clearly see the rotation of the ball as it streaks toward the plate. You feel the looseness and extension

Peak-performance focus and slump focus.

of each stroke and your body riding high in the water, which lets you know your form is perfect and you're going fast. As you bring the ball up the court on a fast break, you can see your teammates filling the wings, racing toward the basket, and know at the last instant who's open to get your pass. When you're in the experience, you pay attention to what's important in the play happening right now and completely block out everything irrelevant. This concentration on the unfolding action is called a "process focus" (see Principle #3, page 5).

In every slumping performance, on the other hand, the athletes' focus of concentration is split. While they try to keep their attention in the experience, they are continually drawn "upstairs" to their thoughts. Simply put, *slumping athletes' attention is always focused in their heads.* Their thinking, internal coaching, and self-criticizing dominate their concentration and get them into trouble time and time again. The lacrosse player runs up the field, thinking, "I'm not getting the job done today *again*. I've gotta start playing better—my opponent is killing me. I know I'm letting the team down." This "head focus" characterizes a slump. This athlete unknowingly distracts himself from the flow of the game with this negative running commentary, which undercuts his confidence, physically slows him down, and causes him to try too hard.

To summarize, when you're in a slump, you pay attention to all the *wrong* things at the *worst* possible times. As the starter calls runners to the line, you question your own training, convinced that your top competitors will go faster because their training was superior to yours. While you await the judge's signal before the start of your floor routine, you worry about mistiming the rotation of your double-back. How badly could you get hurt if you overrotate? The what-ifs steal your courage and kill your confidence.

When you focus properly, your performance world is a wonderful place. Your concentration allows you to relax, have fun, and perform to your potential. (See Principles #1 and #7, pages 4 and 6.) As an athlete, you feel expansive and can't wait for the games to begin. When your focus is off, however, your performance world becomes a harsh, unforgiving, and virtually uninhabitable place. You dread your upcoming performance and can't wait for it to be over. You feel tight. If only you hadn't gotten out of bed that morning.

The Here-and-Now Rule of Peak Performance

If you're stuck in a slump, then learning to consistently focus on the current action of the competition is the next important step toward unlocking your performance. The best way to do this is by understanding and using the here-and-now rule for peak performance. Simply stated, this rule says that to get the most out of practice and perform to your potential when you compete, you must mentally stay in the here and now of these performances. When you're "on" and "in the zone" in competition, you are automatically concentrating on the flow of the action. However, when you're "off" and struggling, you're violating this mental rule. Your head is *everywhere else* except in the here and now.

As a coach, helping your athletes understand this principle is critical to getting them unstuck. Coaching with the here-and-now rule in mind will shorten the duration of their performance difficulties and toughen them mentally. If you violate the here-and-now rule in your coaching, you'll inadvertently undermine your effectiveness.

Time

Concentration has two dimensions: *time* and *place*. When you practice or compete, you can mentally be in one of three "time zones": the past, present, or future. If you're *in the past*, your mind is *behind* your body—your body is performing now, but your mind is dwelling on something that previously occurred. For example, while you perform, your focus could be on a recent mistake, bad call, or missed opportunity. If you're *in the present*, your concentration and your body are *in sync*. Your focus is locked onto what you are doing at that moment. You watch the play as it develops to instinctively determine your next move, see *this* ball coming at you, feel the looseness of the bat in your hands as the pitch is delivered; or run toward the high bar, concentrating on your approach and then, at the perfect moment, switching your focus to your takeoff. If you're *in the future*, your mind is *ahead* of your body as you perform. You're thinking that unless you sink both of these free throws, your team will lose, or you're worrying that you may get lost in the middle of your back tuck as you begin your tumbling pass.

To bust that slump and reach your potential as an athlete, you must learn to consistently stay in the now of your practices and performances. Choking in sports is all about being in the wrong time zone. Successful coaches know this and understand the critical principle of peak performance involved here: focus on the *process*, not the *outcome*. These coaches do not distract their athletes with outcome or future thoughts, such as, "This is a big game, a must-win situation for us" or "If we lose today. . . ." UCLA coaching legend John Wooden always coached the process, not the outcome. Wooden never focused his players on winning, an uncontrollable. Instead, he got them to pay attention to giving a full effort and executing to the best of their ability. In doing so, he narrowed his players' concentration to the process of the game. To be a slump-busting coach, you must actively keep your athletes in the now of the contest.

A personally painful example of leaving the now focus occurred during the finals of my conference championship against a player who had easily defeated me in a dual match during the regular season. Being "on" that day and playing in the now, one point at a time, I was unstoppable. I won the first set 6–3 and plowed my way to a 5–2 lead in the second and final set. I was now about to serve and just four points away from the match and title. As we changed sides, I briefly glanced off the court and noticed an awards table being set up beside the bleachers. Thoughts of glory began to happily dance in my head. I could feel the weight of the winner's trophy in my eager hands. I imagined what it would be like to return to my campus as the conference champion. I had left the now of my match and was basking in the celebration of the future. I became too eager to win and started trying too hard. For the first time all match, I lost my serve. Suddenly, I began to think about how this guy had beaten me in our last match. This past focus made me even more uptight, and my game became tentative. "What if it happened again?" I wondered. I mentally traveled back and forth from the past to the future the rest of the match as I watched my championship and all that imagined glory painfully slip away.

To bust that slump and reach your potential as an athlete, you must learn to consistently stay in the now of your practices and performances.

Thankfully, I had another opportunity to redeem myself the following year. In that match I did no time traveling and kept myself in the now of the performance right through my winning of the championship point. I made sure that I mentally stayed out of the past, a trap that ensnares even the best.

Many slumping athletes and teams carry their past failures and setbacks around with them. The burden of this outdated mental baggage ultimately sinks the performance. Is this what was going on for speed skater Dan Jansen after first falling in the 500 meter sprints in the 1988 Winter Olympics, an event in which he held the world record? Distraught after the death of his sister just before this race, Jansen finished a disappointing fourth in the 1992 Olympics and slipped right before the finish in 1994. He never won that gold medal.

Are the Red Sox carrying around the weight of their one-out-from-victory collapse in the 1978 World Series? Certainly the media would like us to believe that this is exactly what the Buffalo Bills are doing whenever they show up on Super Bowl Sunday, finishing second four years in a row. Are the Buffalo players going onto the field with this past on their minds, or have the sportswriters created this myth of "Super Losers"?

Anytime an athlete or team talks about being cursed by bad luck, they are mentally holding onto the past as they prepare to compete. While the fickle gods of fate certainly play a role in sports, you create or maintain your own bad luck with a past focus. "Here we go again!" "This always happens!" and "Whenever..." are signals that the athlete or team is weighed down by the baggage of the past. Unless you finally decide to let go of the past before you perform, you'll continue to get exactly what you don't want. We will discuss the negative beliefs and thoughts caused by such a focus in more detail in Step 5, "Expecting Success."

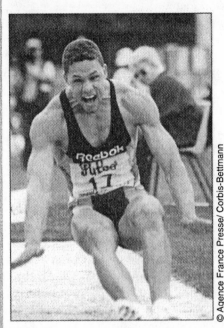

Even the greatest athlete in the world will crumble if his focus is in his head at the wrong time. Witness what a faulty focus did to decathlete Dan O'Brien at the 1992 U.S. Olympic Trials. O'Brien was the reigning world champion, a shoe-in to make the U.S. team and the undisputed favorite to bring back a gold medal from Barcelona. Before the trials, he and David Johnson, another world-class decathlete, had become household names through a series of humorous advertisements for a leading sports company. The burning question posed by the company's ads was, "Who will be the greatest? Dan or Dave? Stay tuned for the Barcelona games where the best athlete in the world will be crowned."

© Agence France Presse/ Corbis-Bettmann

After a couple of successful practice jumps in the pole vault, the eighth event at the trials, O'Brien opened the competition with the bar at 15 feet, 9 inches, a height he'd started with in all of his previous meets. On his first try, O'Brien's perception was thrown off by an unfamiliar pit setup, and he came down hard on the bar. The same thing happened on his second jump, and suddenly O'Brien began to panic. He thought, "I'm down to my last jump. My whole decathlon is on the line. What would people say if I didn't make the team? How would that look?" He began to focus on "not messing up and looking bad." This concentration doomed him. On his third and final jump, he didn't even get up to bar level and "no-heighted" his way off the Olympic team and into the annals of great chokes in sport. The irony of O'Brien's collapse was that he only needed to pole vault 9 feet, 6 inches to make the team!

Fortunately for O'Brien, this humiliating and highly publicized collapse didn't lead to a performance slump or drive him from the sport. He was able to refocus his concentration to rebound from this heartbreak. Several weeks after Czech Robert Zmelik won Olympic gold, O'Brien came back to regain his number 1 world ranking, set a world record, and beat Zmelik by 547 points in an invitational meet in France. Over the next three years, O'Brien established himself as the most prolific decathlete in history and a favorite to win the gold in 1996 in Atlanta. With a new capacity for mental toughness that he developed with the help of a sport psychologist from the U.S. track and field team, he had reinstated his dominance of the sport. O'Brien went on to win the U.S. Trials and, a month later, a gold medal at the Olympic Games.

Had he not redirected his focus, O'Brien, like a lot of athletes before him, could have seen his athletic career fall apart after 1992. He could have taken his humiliation at the 1992 trials, a *past* focus, and carried it with him into all his subsequent meets. In the 1996 trials, he could have used this past failure to choke his way off the team by concentrating on the future with thoughts like, "What if it happened again?" Instead, O'Brien mentally refocused on the here and now of his performance and blocked out irrelevant past failures.

The concept of being in the now as you perform is very basic and something that athletes and coaches frequently overlook because of its simplicity. Yet performing in the wrong time zone can sabotage the performance of even the most talented and well-prepared athlete. Several years ago a world-class swimmer lost 12 50-meter sprints in a row over a year's time after leading in the first 40 meters of each race. She consistently finished these races in the third or fourth position! At the 40-meter mark, her mechanics broke down and her stroke shortened. We traced her problem to a simple time-zone shift at this point in the race. She would inadvertently "leave her body" and jump ahead to the finish, wondering whether she'd be able to finally *win* one or if everyone would catch her *again*. This future focus caused her to tighten up physically and slow down.

It is absolutely critical that you learn to recognize what time zone you're mentally in *before* and *during* your performances. This awareness will help you head off disaster. Knowing, for example, that you tend to dwell on your past mistakes will help you recognize this disruptive time-zone shift and return your concentration to the now of the performance. If you spend several practices working on increasing your awareness of time zones and quickly returning your focus to the proper time as needed, then you'll begin to notice yourself doing this automatically when it counts in competition. Keep in mind that the basis for developing slump-busting concentration and mental toughness is the ability to quickly recognize mental time traveling and immediately bring yourself back to the now of the performance.

As a coach, your awareness of mental time zones will help you get the most out of your athletes and teams. It will insure that your precompetition talks are effective in focusing your athletes in a performance-enhancing way. By keeping your athletes concentrating in the now and by recognizing and stopping their time traveling, you will disrupt their performance difficulties and foster mental toughness.

There is really nothing complex or mysterious that fuels a slump. It's not necessary for you to spend 15 years on a psychologist's couch, unraveling your childhood to find the solution. Slumps rarely involve deep-seated fears of success or failure. They have nothing to do with hidden weaknesses or "holes" in your personality. Leaving the now of the performance is the primary catalyst behind most slumps. Learn to stay in the now, and you'll more consistently be at your best. Leave the now, and your performance will suffer. The now is the only time zone in which you have *complete* access to your skills and training. Furthermore, it is the only time zone that you can directly control. You can't hit hard, run fast, score a goal, or sink that shot when your mind is lagging behind or jumping ahead of your body.

Place

The second dimension of concentration, place, refers to *where* you are mentally as you perform. Not only must you be focused on the right time, but you must also be in the right place. As you step up to take that penalty kick, are you thinking about how good the opposing keeper is? Are you watching the fans waving bright red towels and holding up their "air ball" and "choke" signs as you step to the charity stripe to shoot those clutch free throws? As you move down the field, do you wonder what the coach thinks of your play? Are you preoccupied with those scouts in the stands? Are you worrying about what your boyfriend or girlfriend thinks of you after that mistake? If your answer to any of these questions is yes, then you were in the wrong mental place as you competed. To play to your potential, you must learn to keep yourself in the right mental place, the "here." Let me illustrate this concept of mental place with the following scenario of a college soccer player.

Jola couldn't believe the "no-call." She felt that the refs had been blind all game, calling fouls that didn't exist and letting hard contact go on without the whistle. It was obvious to her that they were favoring the home team. But getting tackled that hard by her opponent without a yellow card or even a lousy whistle was just too much! It was simply unacceptable! She'd seen better officiating when she was playing midget soccer as an eight-year-old. As she quickly picked herself up and ran after the ball, her mind stayed with the officials. She was frustrated and angry. How could the soccer federation allow this? It was outrageous incompetence. As she tried to concentrate, her opponent beat her to a ball, faked her out of her shoes, and took off upfield on a solo run. Jola tried to run her down, but it was too late. As one of Jola's defensive backs came over to help, her opponent hit a centering pass to a wide-open striker, who crushed the ball into the back of the net for the score.

Where was Jola when her team really needed her? Mentally, she was refereeing the game. Her team was one player short while Jola took this leave of absence to evaluate the officiating. Not being in the right mental place prevented her from being in the right tactical place and cost her team a goal, possibly even the match.

When you're not in the here of the performance, it's almost impossible to play to your potential. Furthermore, you are far more vulnerable to the opposition's intimidation. Whether your opponent is deliberately trying to get into your head or not, to get psyched out, *you* must leave the here and focus on *them*.

A swim coach recently took her 17-year-old daughter Katie to the Olympic Trials. A strong, usually confident swimmer, Katie had qualified in the 200-meter breaststroke for the first time. When she got on deck for her first warm-up, she looked around the pool at the IUPUI (Indiana University/Purdue University at Indianapolis) Natatorium, and her eyes got as large as saucers. She began pointing out to her mother with a sense of awe all of the top swimmers whose pictures had graced her swim magazines. She couldn't believe she was actually going to swim against them.

Instead of jumping in the pool and beginning her warm-up, she tentatively asked her mother what lane she should go in. Her mother remarked to me that she hadn't heard that question from her daughter since the girl was a seven-year-old beginner. When her mother suggested that it really didn't matter what lane she warmed up in, Katie seemed immobilized. Finally her mother suggested a specific lane, and Katie's response was that if she went in that lane, she might get "run over" by the other swimmers. There was no question that Katie was intimidated, her worry reflecting the concerns of a seven-year-old, not those of an Olympic Trials qualifier!

Katie was mentally in the wrong place. Her focus of attention was on all the great swimmers around her. When it was time for her to swim, she couldn't help but feel completely out of place. Distracted by *who* was in her heat and how fast they were, she was mentally miles away from the here of her performance. Consequently, her race time was almost five seconds slower than it had been all year. Unfortunately for her, Katie didn't pick up on her mental mistake until her shot at making the Olympic team was gone.

If the athlete, coach, or team catches this mental mistake of leaving the here soon enough, the intimidation can be turned around before it's too late. This happened to a local high school basketball team when it had to play the defending state champions in the first round of the playoffs. Known all around the state as a powerhouse, this girl's team had gone undefeated the previous year to win the title. Despite the fact that the team had lost several key players, it still struck terror into the hearts of opponents. In the first half, the local team played intimidated basketball. The players couldn't stop focusing on *who* they were playing. They turned the ball over 14 times, forced their shots, and couldn't execute plays they had used effectively all season. They missed everything they tried from three-point range and shot

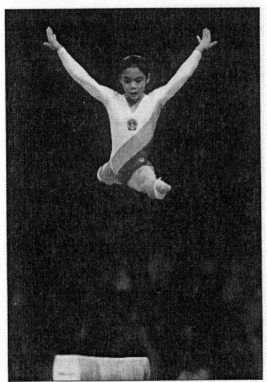

only 23 percent from the field. By halftime they were down by 23 points. They had spent the entire first half in the wrong mental place.

I can only guess what their coach said to them during the break, because in the second half an entirely different group of young women showed up on the court. They focused on *their* game and probably played their best half of basketball all season. They battled their opponents for everything, executed perfectly, and clawed their way back to tie the game at the buzzer, sending it into overtime. They con-

© Claus Andersen

tinued their confident play right through the overtime period, only to lose on a last-second desperation shot. However, despite the loss, they walked off the court having played their game and feeling like winners because of it.

Being psyched out isn't just reserved for athletes and teams. Coaches even fall into this trap. On a recent trip to the Olympic Training Center in Colorado Springs, I had an opportunity to watch several coaches so in awe of their surroundings that they unknowingly had gotten caught up in proving themselves. The coaches were at the OTC with their swimmers for a weekend training clinic. As part of this clinic, they had the opportunity to work daily with their athletes in the U.S. swimming facility. While Olympic-caliber swimmers from the resident team trained under the watchful eyes of the national team coaches, the newcomers began to step outside their normal behavior. One who never yelled began screeching at his swimmer. Another gave his swimmer an uncharacteristically brutal series of sets to do. It was clear to me from the way they looked around that these coaches were intimidated. They couldn't have been in the here of their coaching. They acted as if their coaching competence were being evaluated by the national team staff, who were so involved in their own work that they didn't even notice the new coaches.

There are times, however, when your difficulty staying in the here of the performance is directly related to the extra "help" you may be getting from your opponent. No doubt the opposition's disruptive behavior can knock you off center and adversely affect your play. Whether this is deliberate "gamesmanship" or not, the result is the same. Tennis great John McEnroe was well known for his match-stopping tirades. Whether he thought the linesman was blind or a fan was moving when he shouldn't, Mac would fly off the handle and let his emotions rule the moment. McEnroe frequently came back after these outbursts with renewed intensity, while many of his opponents would fall apart. While John claimed that his emotionality on the court was related to his own frustrations with his poor play and simply a way for him to get back into the match, many of his opponents thought he was doing this to deliberately upset them.

By learning to stay in the right mental place, you can minimize the psychological impact that your opponent's size, strength, speed, record, reputation, or behavior has on you. As a coach, you can neutralize the effects of opponents' mind games by keeping your athletes in the here of the competition, focusing on *their* game, *their* job. Remember, no one can be intimidated unless they agree to it. Leaving the here of the performance and focusing on anyone outside yourself is the only way that you can become vulnerable to this mental trap.

Staying in the Here and Now

Why is being in the here and now so important to slump busting? It's only when you're focusing in the here and now that you are able to automatically respond to the cues necessary for peak performance. When your mind is quiet and focused, your athletically trained senses of sight, touch, and hearing are able to function accurately, zooming in on the ball, opponent, apparatus, or muscle feeling to get the job done. Dribbling by an opponent and beating the goalkeeper, executing a flawless sand shot, throwing a touchdown pass in heavy traffic, or spiking the ball for a winner all require unconscious attention to minimal cues in the environment. For example, when a batter is "on," he's automatically processing the pitcher's stance, motion, release point, and repertoire of pitches, along with the looseness of his own muscles, bat position, good swing mechanics, and timing. Factored in here are the weather conditions and their effect on the ball, the size of the strike zone as called by this umpire, and the muscle memories of that just-right swing from thousands of past at-bats. This is all done unconsciously with an "empty mind" as the batter loosens his arms and narrows his focus of concentration to the ball.

It's only when you're focusing in the here and now that you are able to automatically respond to the cues necessary for peak performance.

When this same athlete slumps, he's "in his head," either in the past or future, or in the wrong mental place. As a result, he will likely miss some of these internal and external performance cues needed to get the job done. Too much "noise" in his head distracts him, throwing his timing and execution off just enough to create negative results. Rather than relaxing and returning his focus to the proper cues, the struggling batter starts looking for a solution. Unfortunately, he almost always looks in the wrong place. He makes too many changes or thinks too much about his grip, stance, swing mechanics, or bat position when there is no problem here. He worries about his falling average and keeps track of how many games he's gone without hitting the ball out of the infield. He thinks, "I gotta get a hit" when he's at the plate instead of letting go and trusting himself. He's mentally out to lunch instead of in the here and now. One failure leads to another as his frustration mounts.

How do you get yourself back in the here and now where *all* the solutions to your performance problems lie? First, you have to learn to recognize when you leave the right time and place. Second, you have to quickly and gently bring yourself back to the proper focus within the here and now. Coaches can help their athletes do this by directly assigning them specific places on which to lock their concentration. Let me give you an example from the athlete's perspective.

Jamal was a talented high school ballplayer who had been struggling with his hitting all season. One of the best hitters on his squad, he had almost no tolerance for his string of lousy at-bats. However, like all slumping athletes, the more frustrated he got with his failures, the more he failed. Jamal was a statistician at heart, and it was this preoccupation with his numbers and "production" that was keeping him stuck. Jamal knew he had to relax and stay in the here and now of each at-bat. He knew he must not take his bad at-bats onto the field with him. However, knowing these things intellectually and actually doing them were two different things. Jamal was having trouble controlling his self-directed rage at his perceived incompetence.

Then Jamal hit on a brilliant idea. I had assured him that the moment he was able to consistently stay loose at the plate, his hitting would return to normal. He thought, "What if I switch my statistics-keeping at the plate from the results of each at-bat (a future or outcome focus) to how relaxed I am, both before and after each hit (a process focus)?" Instead of keeping a batting average, he would now keep a "relaxing average" (here-and-now focus). If Jamal could *feel looseness* in his arms, hands, and legs as well as feel a *smile* on his face before and during his first at-bat, he would be 1 for 1 according to his relaxing average, *regardless of whether he got a hit*. If he was thinking about getting a hit or worrying about his coach or the pitcher, he would receive an 0 for 1 for this at-bat, whether he hit or not. Similarly, if he stayed relaxed and left the previous at-bat in the past, his "average" would be 2 for 2. Jamal's idea helped him to shift himself back into the experience of the here and now. His new focus enabled him to pay attention to the proper cues again. Soon he was going 2 for 4 in his "relaxing average" and starting to hit again. In a recent game, he came to the plate with two outs and the winning run on base. In the past, this chance for glory would have gotten into his head and knocked him out of the here and now. He would have stepped to the plate trying too hard and thinking, "Yeah, chance to be a hero!" and "They'll write me up for this one!" Instead, he focused on his "relaxing average," loosening his hands, shoulders, arms, and legs. He drove a hard single up the middle to win the game.

Controlling Your Eyes and Ears

Besides developing first an awareness of when you leave the here and now and then the ability to quickly bring yourself back, what do you actually do to stay in the right mental time and place? Controlling your eyes and ears before and during competition is the answer. Before and during a game, you should *look* at and *listen* to only those things that keep you calm, confident, and ready to perform to your potential. The high jumper who stares at the ground two minutes before his turn, the free-throw shooter who focuses on the rim before her shot, and the rower who stares at a spot in the middle of his teammate's back as he rows are all controlling their eyes. The soccer player who listens to his favorite tape before the game, the wrestler who pumps himself up by telling himself everything he's done to prepare, and the triathlete who listens to the sound of her footstrike as she runs are all controlling their ears.

Athletes who have difficulty controlling their eyes and ears before or during performance invariably run into repeated performance problems. The inability to control your focus is what causes most slumps and keeps them running. By learning to control *where* you focus your eyes and ears *before* and *during* performance, you will be well on your way to busting that slump.

> **B**y learning to control where you focus your eyes and ears before and during performance, you will be well on your way to busting that slump.

Preperformance.   Wandering eyes mean a wandering mind and frequently a slump-feeding, self-destructive focus. Controlling your eyes entails locking your visual focus of attention on specific, prearranged points *before* your performance. Where you focus your eyes is especially important when there is a natural stoppage in the flow of the performance, such as a timeout, a break between halves, or time between races, events, or shots. It is during these nonplaying times when you have plenty of time to think that you're most vulnerable to a performance-disrupting loss of focus. As in all sports, the more time you have to get into your head, the more creative ways you'll discover to set yourself up for failure.

Controlling your eyes *preperformance* means that in the hours, minutes, and seconds before competition starts, you look only at things that keep you calm, loose, and confident. "Preperformance" also includes the times just before you go to the foul line for that one-and-one, in between preliminaries and the final heat, the walk to your next golf shot, and those few minutes before you go out to take that kick in the sudden-death shootout. In short, you have to learn to control what you look at *any time* there is a break in the action and the flow is about to restart.

If focusing your attention on friends pre-event helps keep you centered, then continue doing this. If looking into the stands or at your opponents makes you uptight, *don't* do it. Instead, find somewhere else to deliberately focus your eyes. Reading a book before or between events, watching your legs as you stretch them, picking out one spot and staring at it, looking down at your shoes, and focusing on your glove are all examples of what you can do to control your eyes. By picking specific targets to look at ahead of time and regularly using them, you'll have a much easier time successfully staying calm and confident when it counts. These visual targets or focal points will distract you from the real distractions.

> **C**ontrolling your eyes preperformance means that before competition starts you look only at things that keep you calm, loose, and confident.

Using the same focal points repeatedly will contribute to your comfort and confidence, because anything familiar tends to neutralize anxiety. It's the unfamiliar that causes athletes to get too anxious to play to their potential. The first time qualifying for state, competing in the Junior Olympics, or making it to the Final Four or to your conference Super Bowl naturally generates fear and anxiety along with excitement. Because of your emotions in these situations, you're more vulnerable to losing your focus. Having a familiar target for your eyes in these new and highly stressful situations will minimize your chances of choking.

Sport psychologist Ken Ravizza from Cal State-Fullerton teaches athletes a technique to help them master these new situations and use focal points to their advantage. In 1984 Ken worked with the U. S. field hockey team in helping them prepare for the Los Angeles Olympics. The team, comprised of athletes from around the country, ran their practices on the very field where the Olympics would be held. While many of the team members had never played before an audience bigger than a few hundred, the seating capacity of this stadium was many thousands. To help them control their eyes and ears, Ken had them "make friends with the field." This entailed walking around the empty field and stadium, getting comfortable with it, and picking out two or three focal points that they knew would be there once competition began and the place was rocking.

Often, thinking about where *not* to focus can hinder performance. Self-coaching, such as, "She's right next to you—don't look at her," "That crowd is so big—don't look over there," and "Don't think about how strong he is" only serves to keep athletes focused on all the wrong things. When you tell yourself *not* to look at something, the looking continues in your mind's eye. Having a specific visual target for your eyes enables you to control your attention in a more constructive way.

Good coaching can help athletes control their visual focus. As a coach, teach your athletes the *right* things to focus on preperformance, not the wrong ones. If you've told them exactly what they should be concentrating on before the game starts, they'll be more likely to recognize when they lose that focus and will know automatically where to refocus.

Like controlling your eyes, controlling your ears entails listening to only those things that keep you calm, confident, and ready to perform your best. To control your ears, you must learn to monitor two sources of auditory input: sounds coming from *outside* yourself, for example, the crowd, a teammate, or a trash-talking opponent; and sounds coming from *inside* yourself, your self-talk. Spend as little time as possible listening to things that drain your confidence. Instead, substitute positive or neutral sounds that will distract you from the negatives. (In Step 5, "Expecting Success," we will address techniques you can use to neutralize negative self-talk and replace it with positive self-talk.) Many athletes control their ears by listening to music before the performance. Others repeat specific affirmations to themselves before they perform. For example, one high school runner repeated to herself "P, C, P" (powerful, confident, positive) before the start of each race to neutralize her tendency to think about her opponents' strengths, question her own skill, and wallow in the negative. The "P, C, P" helped counteract her habitual negative mind-set and reminded her of the right focus while simultaneously neutralizing her old self-doubts and negativity.

> *L*earn to monitor both sounds coming from outside yourself and sounds coming from inside yourself.

Using the Preperformance Ritual. To systematically control your eyes and ears and stay in the here and now, develop a set preperformance ritual or routine. Every great athlete has one and uses it to stay focused and confident before the action starts. The pitcher on the mound, free-throw shooter at the line, golfer over the ball, and tennis player getting ready to serve all have a routine that helps them narrow their concentration and prepare for successful execution. This routine can be elaborate or simple. It can begin a half-hour or more before a performance or just a few seconds before it. It can involve saying certain things to yourself, a quick mental rehearsal, repeating specific behaviors, or some combination of all of these.

A good ritual keeps athletes centered and focused in the here and now of the performance just before it begins. It keeps their minds off all the potential distractions and stressors within the competitive environment. The ritual provides them with a systematic way to gradually narrow their focus, so that when the action begins, they have perfect one-point concentration.[1] The narrowing process is accomplished through paying attention to the focal points within the ritual.

A good ritual keeps athletes centered and focused in the here and now of the performance just before it begins.

Team rituals function much the same way. They keep the athletes as a group relaxed and focused. When playing an away game in a hostile environment where everything is unfamiliar, the team's ritual during the day, on the bus ride over, and during pregame warm-up becomes a safe port in a storm for the athletes—something they can control that is comfortable and familiar.

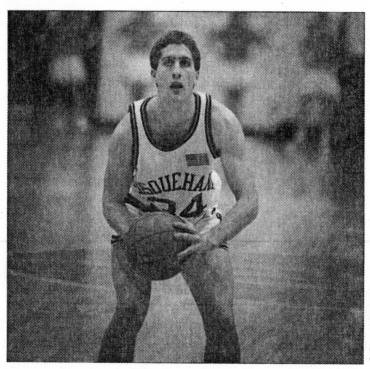

© Terry Wild Studio

Figure 3.1 illustrates the process of narrowing concentration before the performance. Well before the action begins, your concentration can be very broad (left side of the diagram). You can be thinking any number of things that may or may not be related to the upcoming performance. Whatever works for you—thoughts about Hawaii, pepperoni pizza, or Saturday night's planned party—will fit here, as will another athlete's regular pregame analysis of his opponent's strategy. As the time of the performance approaches, however, you need to leave Hawaii and mentally start to narrow your concentration. Your ritual or routine provides the vehicle to effectively narrow your focus of concentration as the competition approaches, culminating in a single focus point as the performance begins.

Let's say, for example, that you're a basketball player who will be going to the line to shoot two clutch free throws. The opposing team's coach called a full timeout just before your shots to give you plenty of time to contemplate all the potential consequences of failure. You have about 30 seconds before you step out there and face those screaming fans hoping to

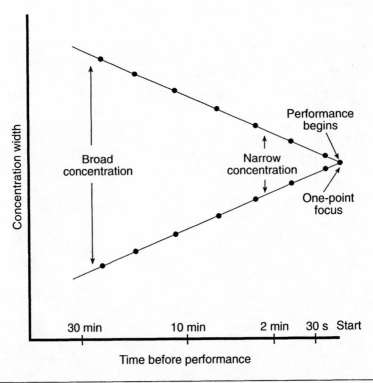

Figure 3.1 Narrowing concentration before performance (each dot on the graph represents a focal point of the preperformance ritual).

distract you. If there ever was a time that you needed to control your eyes and ears, this is it. Your mind seems to be all over the place. Thoughts of fame and fortune that will result *if* you make them both dance in your head. You remember three games ago when the team let the coach down by losing in overtime. You wonder why you're thinking about that now, when you suddenly realize the coach has been talking and is looking directly at you. The buzzer sounds and the timeout ends. You get off the bench and head for the foul line. As you do, all of the fans in the gym jump up yelling "air ball."

You slowly narrow your concentration by doing what you always do before taking a free throw. This preshot ritual might resemble the following:

You walk to the top of the key looking only at the back of the rim. When you reach the line, you stop and, like Larry Bird, rub the bottom of each shoe with the opposite hand—first the left hand for the right foot, and then the right hand for the left foot. As you walk to the line and the ref hands you the ball, you switch your focus down to the charity stripe and line up your toes exactly one inch behind it. Next you pick a spot right in front of you and bounce the ball four times, trying to hit that spot. Then you look at the ball and rotate it in your hands until you have it in your favorite position—writing up, facing you, lined up perfectly. You take a slow deep breath and pick out your target spot on the rim. Then, very slowly and quietly, you repeat the word "swish" to yourself three times, hearing that familiar sound in your head as you do so. You feel your knees bend and then simply let the ball fly through the net.

Each little step in your preshot ritual had a purpose: to capture your attention and keep both the fans and the situation from getting into your head. Every familiar step in the routine narrowed your concentration and helped you empty your mind until you shot. Such a preperformance ritual is effective only if you stay in the here and now as you go through it. In other words, you must do what you are doing *mentally* while you are doing it *physically*. A ritual will not narrow your focus if your mind is not on what you're doing. If as you stretch prerace as you always do, you focus on your opponent's strength, your stretching ritual is useless. While you may see preperformance rituals in slumping athletes, you will not find their minds attached to what they are doing.

A word of caution here. Keep your rituals short and simple. Be sure that they involve things that are easy for you to do and don't depend on outside elements that you might not be able to control. You *can always* control stretching in a set pattern, repeating certain phrases to yourself, focusing on and checking your equipment in a familiar way, and jumping up and down before the contest. You *can't always* control having other people say or do certain things to you, eating a special pregame meal, having exactly one hour to warm up, or having your favorite bat available (what if it breaks in the middle of the game?). Remember the ritual's purpose—to help you stay calm and focused and in control, *not* make you feel out of control.

During Performance. If a ritual or single focal point helps you control your eyes and ears *before* the performance, what do you do to stay in the here and now *during* the performance? In many sports, your major during-performance focal point is the ball or puck. However, frequently your focus may also have to partially or completely shift to a defensive or offensive task away from the puck or ball. For example, as an offensive lineman in football, your job is to focus on the oncoming rusher and block him out of the play. In basketball and soccer, you must focus on moving without the ball in anticipation of getting it. In hockey, you may have to focus on physically tying up your opponent so that he can't execute.

Always lock your attention on a focal point during breaks in the action. Tennis players fiddle with their strings, batters look down at the dirt, and pitchers stare at the ball to help keep their minds from wandering to potential distractions. However, in many sports where action is more continuous and there isn't a puck or ball to hold attention, the athletes must find other ways to hold their attention when it starts to leave the here and now of the performance.

In any kind of race, for example, you must be able to continuously lock your attention on specific internal and external cues that help you maintain a proper pace. You may concentrate on the *feeling* of staying loose and long with your stroke as a swimmer, pulling hard into the feeling of pain with each stroke you take in your boat, or the rhythm of your footstrike as you run. In these sports, however, it is quite easy for your mind to wander during the race. When this happens and you stop paying attention to the cues that make you go fast, you begin to lose valuable time. To counteract this natural tendency, you must develop specific during-race focal points that you can return your attention to immediately after you've recognized that you've strayed from the here and now of the experience.

For example, Tim was a swimmer with a bad habit of focusing on what was going on in the lanes around him. At meets, this preoccupation distracted him from his own race and slowed him down. Unlike some athletes who can motivate themselves by watching and thinking about their opponents, Tim would use this outside focus to self-destruct. His coach had told him numerous times to "swim in your own lane" and forget about everyone else, but Tim seemed unable to control his focus in the heat of competition. When he swam his fastest, Tim's race focus was on the *feeling* of pulling water with his arms. When he began looking around and thinking about his opponents, Tim would stop feeling his arms and therefore slow down.

Then his coach came up with the idea to paint red dots on the sides of his goggles, so that if Tim glanced sharply left or right, he'd catch a glimpse of red. The coach explained that the color red meant two things. First, it signified all the hard work that Tim had put into training. It was a reminder that he had paid his physical dues and belonged in the pool with anybody. Second, the color red symbolized what it does the world over, "Stop!" The coach explained that when Tim glanced to his side during a race and saw that color, he would immediately remember these two meanings and refocus on the feeling of pulling in his arms.

As a cyclist, swimmer, runner, rower, or triathlete, where are you most vulnerable in the race? Do you tend to forget your race plan and go out too fast because of a focus on the competition? Do you lose it mentally when a particular opponent passes you? Is there a specific part of the race when you usually hit the wall and get negative? Find these places of vulnerability where your mind leaves the here and now of the race and develop focal points to help you get through them. When you run into these challenging parts of the competition, you need to have something positive and constructive on which to focus your concentration.

When you run into challenging parts of the competition, you need to have something positive and constructive on which to focus your concentration.

For example, let's say that as a distance runner, you tend to lose it mentally when you get passed by certain opponents. In the past, your reflex reaction to seeing their backsides was to start putting yourself down and completely forgetting about your race strategy. As a consequence of this negativity, you'd become overly preoccupied with how tired you felt, physically tighten up, and then slow down. Ideally in these situations, you should keep focused on *your* race and maintain your looseness and pace. One focal point that you can deliberately go to whenever you get passed is that familiar and comfortable feeling of physical looseness in your stride. You may instead shift to the easy rhythm breathing or feel of your arm swing. You can even use that old negative self-talk about being left behind as a cue to get yourself right back to that loose feeling in your legs or these other performance cues. At this point in the run, you may also use a verbal reminder—"my race"—to help you maintain your composure, stay within yourself, and run your own race.

Scott was a freshman placekicker for a small-college football team. In high school he was a standout who could kick with accuracy from 40 yards. He had successfully kicked the point after touchdown (PAT) in 37 consecutive high school games, a conference record. He continued this excellence into the three games of freshman pre-season—then everything seemed to fall apart in his first college season start. His first PAT was blocked and then he badly missed a 20-yard field goal attempt. In his next attempt, with the game on the line, his team down by two and the ball on the opponent's 15-yard line, Scott lined up the potential game winner. As he approached the ball, he seemed tentative and unsure of himself. What should have been a routine kick didn't even make the crossbars.

From there things seemed to go from bad to worse. In practice he was distracted by confidence-eroding thoughts that began to haunt him in games. He continued to replay the bad opening game over and over again in his mind's eye. He couldn't seem to shake worries that the past would repeat itself. In games, thoughts like *"What if* I don't hit it hard enough?" *"What if* I don't line it up right?" and *"What if* I don't make this?"* followed him from the sidelines to the huddle. He was distracted enough by these thoughts to continue to struggle. In his second game he missed three out of four PATs and all three field goal attempts.

By the time his coach finally called me, Scott's confidence was at an all-time low and his slump had extended into six games. As he described the problem, I was struck by how much "time traveling" Scott was doing during his games. He was regularly violating the here-and-now rule for peak performance. If he wasn't in the past reviewing recent misses, he was jumping ahead and previewing his next failure. The only time he seemed to be able to keep himself in the now of the performance was when he went out to practice by himself. It was during these times that he could settle himself down to kick like the Scott of old.

Scott's faulty focus seemed to be the main culprit in causing and maintaining his slump. I reasoned that if he could successfully get himself to remain in the now of the performance, his kicking accuracy and consistency would quickly return. I helped him do this by first reviewing in detail every step that he went through in practice and past games when he kicked successfully. In doing this Scott laid out an elaborate pre-kick ritual that he had been unknowingly using to keep himself calm and properly focused. Every step in the ritual utilized *focal points* that helped him *stay in the now and control his eyes and ears.* He realized that in every one of his bad games he had shortened or completely omitted this ritual. His pre-kick ritual was as follows:

1. Determine field position, angle, and wind speed and direction
2. Clear his head and block out distractions by staring at a spot on the ground
3. Stretch his hamstrings in both legs for approximately five seconds
4. Look up at the uprights and narrow his target
5. Place his plant (left) foot down exactly where it should be, paying attention to the *feeling* of his foot
6. Take three normal steps back, counting to himself and feeling his feet on the turf
7. Stand upright, take a deep breath, and slowly let it out
8. Say "ready Freddy" to the signal caller to let him know that he was set

At this point all of his concentration was focused on the holder's hands, where the ball was going to be in a matter of seconds.

By helping Scott stay focused on every step of this ritual in the now of the performance and teaching him how to quickly bring himself back every time his mind wandered, he was able to start making the PATs and field goals again. While he knew intellectually that his concentration had been off, he wasn't doing anything to bring himself back to the now where all his accuracy and consistency resided.

Many athletes use auditory focal points, like a verbal reminder, during a performance to block out other distracting, performance-upsetting noises. One softball pitcher repeats to herself the phrase "loose arms, now target" several times before every pitch. Within this phrase are two important cues that guarantee a fast and accurate pitch: The feeling of looseness in her arms helps her throw fast, and narrowing her focus to the catcher's glove, her primary target for each pitch. By repeating this phrase mantra-like to herself, she is able to drown out the crowd's razzing and remind herself where to lock her concentration.

If you're the kind of athlete who is easily distracted by noise (a trash-talking opponent, rowdy crowd, or plane flying overhead), try developing other sounds (internal or external) that you can focus on to counteract the distractions. These can be certain words that you repeat to yourself, a tune you play in your head, or some specific sound that is always part of your performance (your breathing, the oar movement as you row, the ball bouncing, or your footstrike while running).

Developing Focal Points

How do you decide what focal points *you* should use before and during performance? First, think back to some of your better performances. Can you remember what specifically you focused on right before the performance began (refer to the "What Mental Strategies Are You Using?" exercise in Step 2 on page 28)? Were you listening to music? Talking with friends? Mentally reviewing the upcoming performance? Stretching or warming up and focusing on how your body was feeling? Looking at something specific in the competitive arena? How about during the performance? What were you concentrating on? Was it a kinesthetic or body feeling (a feeling of the movement of your arms or legs as you executed)? Something that you visually locked your eyes on? A particular sound? Some combination of these?

By reviewing past peak performances in this way, you may be able to discover some important clues as to what focal points best help you control your eyes and ears. To further help you do this, think back to some of your poorer performances and try to recall where your focus was for these before and during the action. Can you recall whether you were distracted by something visual ("I couldn't take my eyes off of how tall my opponents were")? Kinesthetic ("I felt so stiff and tight and I kept focusing on how bad I felt")? Auditory ("This one guy kept razzing me every time I stepped up to the line, I couldn't get his voice out of my head")?

As you can see, focal points can be visual, kinesthetic, auditory, or some combination of the three. Based on your review of good and bad performances, can you determine which kind of focal point works best for you? If the size of the crowd or the appearance of your opponents during warmups tends to upset you, then develop *visual* focal points before the game to counteract those distractions. If negative self-talk, comments from the fans, or an opponent's verbal challenge bother you before the match, then develop *auditory* focal points. Similarly, if feelings of fatigue, stiffness, or low energy tend to fuel your prerace panic, refocus on different *kinesthetic* focal points (such as the feelings of stretching, warming up, or your breathing).

Developing performance focal points entails figuring out where your concentration needs to be to insure optimal execution. By examining your focus during past good performances, you'll discover some of these focal points. Since peak performance is an unconscious process, you may not remember exactly what you were focusing on. Upon closer review, however, you should be able to identify specific visual, kinesthetic, and/or auditory cues that worked for you. For most athletes, focusing on a certain just-right feeling in their body as they perform (kinesthetic cue) leads to peak performance. The diver, gymnast, skater, basketball player, and high jumper all intuitively zero in on a specific kinesthetic focal point when they are at their best. Similarly, many sports demand specific visual focal points (such as the ball, puck, or target) in the action for optimal performance.

D *eveloping performance focal points entails figuring out where your concentration needs to be to insure optimal execution.*

Once you've discovered which focal points seem to work for you, consciously use them daily in practice. For example, when you're exhausted toward the end of a session and feel that strong urge to let your mind wander, bring yourself back to your focal point(s) instead. Use that feeling of fatigue to pick up your pace and loosen your muscles, exactly the way you would want to do if you were in the middle of a race. If negative thinking or fear is setting in before you jump, refocus yourself on the feelings of one part of that jump. Understand that you will consistently compete the way you practice. If you practice successfully handling those vulnerable parts of your competition by quickly and constructively refocusing yourself, you will feel increased confidence the next time you are challenged by them in an actual contest.

As a coach, you can actively teach mental toughness by helping your athletes develop these during-performance focal points and having them regularly practice concentrating on them during training. If you can teach your athletes *where* to focus when they are under physical and competitive stress, and you have them practice controlling their concentration in this way, then they will be far less vulnerable to mental breakdowns in the heat of competition.

Testing Your Concentration Ability

How well do you stay in the here and now of the performance? Is concentration at the heart of your performance difficulties? To answer these questions, try the following exercise.

WHAT DISTRACTS YOU?

Sitting comfortably in a space that's free from distractions, close your eyes and pay attention to your breathing. Your focus can be on the sound of your breathing, the feeling of the rise and fall of your diaphragm, the air coming into and going out from your nose and mouth, an image that connects you to the breathing process such as a wave coming in to and receding from the shore, or any combination of these. While you inhale comfortably and naturally, pay attention to this breathing focal point. As you exhale, switch your focus to the number "one." You may visualize a number one in your mind's eye, repeat the word "one" to yourself, or somehow combine these two. When you first become aware that your mind has left the proper focus, bring yourself back to your breathing and counting, except this time go to the number "two." Focus on your breathing as you inhale and on the number "two" as you exhale. Continue this until you become distracted again, and then shift to the number "three." Each time you become aware of a loss of focus, add a number.

For the first part of this exercise, spend two minutes sitting and counting to yourself. When the two minutes have elapsed, record three items:

1. What was the last number you were focusing on?

2. What did you focus on with each inhalation and exhalation—a visual, auditory, or kinesthetic focal point? For example, did you listen to your breathing and repeat the numbers out loud in your mind? Did you pay attention to the physical feeling of your inhalation and exhalation as you counted? Did you use visual images as focal points, seeing your numbers or an image that accompanied your breathing?

3. When your focus did wander, what caused the distraction? Were you more distracted by sights, sounds, or internal feelings? For example, did you find yourself listening to noises around you or the sound of your inner dialogue? Did you tend to get sidetracked by visual images around the room or in your mind's eye? Did bodily sensations interrupt your concentration?

For the second timed two-minute period of this exercise, play a radio station, tape, or CD you enjoy. Repeat the same exercise, again with your eyes closed, focusing on your breathing as you inhale and the counting as you exhale. Add a number each time you get distracted. When the two minutes have elapsed, record the number you reached; whether your attention was locked on a visual, auditory, kinesthetic, or combination focal point; and what you found distracted you most.

For the third part of this exercise, sit about three feet from a television or directly by an open window with an interesting view. Repeat the two-minute exercise with your eyes open while the TV is on or while looking out the window. Again, record the number you reached, what you chose to focus on as you breathed, and what you found to be the most distracting.

The final part of this exercise involves sitting a few feet away from a fan, air-conditioning unit, or heater. Sitting outside if a strong breeze is blowing or if it's raining (assuming it's relatively warm out) would also work. For the two-minute period, once more with your eyes shut, go through the concentration exercise, attempting to maintain your focal points while you can feel the air, heat, cold, or rain. Once more record the number you ended with, what you found yourself focusing on, and what specifically distracted you most.

Evaluating the Results

Let's take a brief look at your concentration ability, the foundation skill for mental toughness. This exercise involves two concentration subskills. First, it measures, although somewhat crudely, your ability to focus on one thing and block out a series of distractions. Second, it tests your ability to recognize when you've lost your focus and to quickly get back to the target focus. In the first part of this exercise, there were no outward distractions, but there was potential for being knocked off track by inner ones. The second part involved distractions that were primarily auditory or sound-based, while the third and fourth parts used visual- and kinesthetic-based distractions, respectively.

Look at the four numbers you recorded, representing the amount of times that you lost your focus and had to bring yourself back. With what kind of distraction was your number the highest? For example, let's say that in your first two-minute period, you counted to 15, and in the next three periods, you got no higher than 8 in each. This result would indicate that you are more vulnerable to internal "noise," like the chatter of your own self-talk. If your third trial was the highest, visual stimuli tend to throw you off. Compare these numbers with your own experience of what you found most distracting in each trial.

Another way we could score this test and your concentration ability is by looking at the specific number you reached in each part. For example, if you stayed between 1 and 4 throughout each trial, we can make a somewhat fair assumption that your ability to consistently maintain a focus, regardless of the source of distractions, is quite exceptional. If you hovered between 5 and 8 after each two-minute period, we can assume that your concentration ability is somewhat above average. Scores of 9 to 13 are average, and scores between 14 and 17 indicate that you are easily distracted. If you recorded a number 18 or higher, we can conclude that concentration is at the heart of your performance troubles.

If you scored high, however, there's no need to push the panic button. Judging your concentration ability by these numbers is not precise. It is possible for someone with poor concentration skills to record a low number on this test. For example, if you lose your focus as you begin and only wake up at the end of the allotted time period, you can end up with a low number. Similarly, a high number does not necessarily indicate that you can't concentrate. On the contrary, it can also reflect an enhanced awareness of a loss of focus and an above-average ability to quickly return to the target focus.

So if your number in each trial is not totally accurate in judging your focusing ability, how can you constructively evaluate and use the results of this test? The most important thing you can learn from this test is the kinds of distractions that corral your attention and knock you off track. Did you get to a higher number when you faced internal, visual, auditory, or kinesthetic distractions?

Knowing, for example, that you are most susceptible to a break in concentration because of visual distractions can help you strengthen your overall concentration skills. Armed with this information, you can plan ahead to develop a strong defense against visual intrusions before and during performance. This might mean that you build in more visual focal points or "anchors" into your preperformance routine. These visual anchors would then help you prevent your eyes from wandering during those crucial moments just before the start. Also, you could plan during-performance anchors that would help you better control your eyes and stay in the here and now of the action.

This test can also show how you concentrate best. That is, in which sense was it the easiest for you to maintain your focus with the fewest distractions to your concentration? When you focused on your breathing, did you find yourself listening to the *sound* of your inhalation and exhalation while you repeated the numbers loudly in your head? Did the *feeling* of the inhalation and exhalation work better as a way to lock your focus on the task at hand? Did you use some combination of *sound, sight, and feeling* that helped you stay at a low number? Knowing what sense works best for you is critical to maintaining your focus under pressure.

Another useful aspect of this exercise is that with sufficient practice, it will help you strengthen your "concentration muscle." As a two-part skill, concentration is the ability to first recognize when your mind has drifted from the proper focus and then quickly return to it. Consistently practicing this activity with special emphasis on the parts that you found most distracting will help you develop this important mental skill.

Conclusion

Slumps are frequently caused and maintained by a faulty focus of concentration. To bust that slump, you need to learn how to shift your focus of attention from your head to the experience of the action. To do this, you need to consistently integrate the here-and-now rule for peak performance into your practice and competition. By staying in the right mental time and place, and learning to control your eyes and ears before and during performance, you will make great progress toward breaking the slump.

After developing control over your concentration, you will discover that all remaining steps in the slump-busting model become easier to accomplish. Having a championship focus forms the foundation to help you overcome fears, expect success, develop positive images, successfully set slump-busting goals, build self-confidence, become mentally tough, and insure against future slumps.

In the next step, you will learn to face and overcome fears that may be maintaining your slump. By systematically dismantling these fears, you will start to feel like your old performance self again—more confident and in control.

STEP 4

DEALING WITH YOUR FEARS

"Of all the liars in the world, sometimes the worst are your own fears."

—Rudyard Kipling

Fear is at work in most performance slumps. The batter in a slump is afraid of not getting a hit. The gymnast stuck on a round-off, back handspring, or back tuck is afraid of moving backward. The diver stuck on a reverse-and-a-half is terrified of hitting her head on the board. The swimmer who seems to "die" at the end of all her races is afraid of "it" happening again. The pro basketball player who has had trouble making the permanent roster of every team he's tried out for is constantly worried about getting cut once more. For all these athletes, their fears become catalysts that propel them into a slump and keep them stuck there.

To bust that slump and get yourself back on track, you have to face up to these fears and defeat them. Fear tightens your muscles and distracts you from a winning focus. Fear steals the one thing you need as an athlete to excel: your heart. It takes away your nerve, fills your head with worries, and kills your confidence. Fear takes you out of being "in the experience" where peak performance happens and instead puts you "in your head" where absolutely nothing good happens. Furthermore, fear kills your fun, a critical element of peak performance.

In this next step of the slump-busting model, you'll learn how to *recognize* fear's various guises, *understand* the role you may be inadvertently playing in generating your fear, and *take action* to neutralize the

75

performance-disrupting effects of the fear. Step 4 will teach you a number of effective fear-busting strategies that will help you continue the process of retrieving your old sense of control and personal power that you started back in Steps 2 and 3 of the model.

The slump-inducing effects of fear can be powerful. For example, in 1989 the New England Patriots picked defensive cornerback Maurice Hurst out of Southern University in the fourth round of the NFL draft. In 1994 he signed a three-year contract worth $5.1 million. He was one more piece in coach Bill Parcells's Super Bowl puzzle that was just beginning to take shape. Parcells considered Hurst to be "the best cover guy I've ever coached." After a rocky start in 1994, Hurst and the Patriots played brilliantly the remainder of the season. Although they lost in the divisional playoffs, Parcells was optimistic that 1995 was going to be the Patriots' year.

What Parcells wasn't counting on was that Hurst, considered by many to be the best coverage cornerback in New England history, picked 1995 to fall into a massive playing slump. Hurst's problems really began that summer in training camp when he developed a herniated disk in his neck. The resulting soreness and "burners" (loss of feeling) shooting down his left arm after hard contact scared him, planting fears about the possibility of paralysis should he continue to play. Hurst carried this fear into the home opener and was beaten twice for two scores. Other coverage problems followed in the next two games, and for the first time in his career Hurst began to question himself. His self-doubts and inability to let go of his fears caused him to play tentatively.

Later in September Hurst's off-season trainer, Mackie Shilstone, a New Orleans professional who works with heavyweight boxer Riddick Bowe, warned Hurst that his condition could lead to paralysis if he continued to play without having it surgically repaired. Not one to make excuses for himself, Hurst continued to play, but his fear and cautiousness led to more uncharacteristic mistakes. Soon he became preoccupied with whether he was going to cost the Patriots the game. "If someone completed a 5-yard slant on me and they went on to score I'd think that play was the turning point, that the team won't regroup. I'd think, 'Now Maurice, they can point the finger at you.'"[1]

Even Hurst knew that mentally his game was in big trouble because of these fears. "I used to never hesitate about what to do. I never used to enter a game thinking about the other guy catching a touchdown on me. If it happened, it happened but I never thought about it until this year. I began to be doubtful. When that happens you're history. It's over once you doubt yourself a little bit."[2]

Like most slumps, Hurst's seemed to gain an unstoppable momentum as the season progressed. In mid-November, after another poor outing, Parcells called Hurst into his office and fired him. Hurst's slump seemed to have started because of his fear of sustaining a more serious injury and was then further fed by fears of poor performance. Because he wasn't able to control his fears, Hurst was never really able to get his head and focus of concentration back on the field where it belonged.

To beat fear, you must learn to return your focus to the competition as it unfolds around you. For example, Sally was a precociously talented soft-ball pitcher with Olympic-caliber potential. As an eighth grader, she could easily hold her own with high school and college athletes. On the mound she had tremendous speed, excellent control, and several good pitches. Her mother called me last year because Sally's game was slumping. She had lost her trademark control and was walking an unusually large number of batters. Her mother mentioned that Sally was no longer confident on the mound and against better hitters seemed downright tentative, even scared. Her mother added that Sally's problems seemed to have started some six months ago when she was hit in the face by a line drive. Luckily

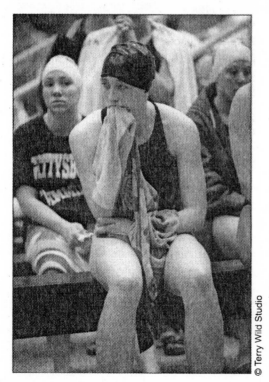
© Terry Wild Studio

the ball didn't do any serious damage physically, but it took a toll on Sally mentally.

Whenever she faced a team that she thought had strong hitters, Sally got tentative and wild. When she faced batters she knew weren't strong, she was able to set her fear aside, relax, and throw hard strikes. As you can easily guess, Sally's problem stemmed directly from her fear-based focus. Against a strong batter, she would think about the possibility of getting hit again. Against a weaker batter, she would pay attention to keeping her arm loose, picking a target, and letting the throw happen. Within the crucial difference in concentration between these two experiences lay the solution to her problem. When she was doing well, her focus was on what she *wanted to happen* and getting the job done. When she struggled, her concentration was locked onto what she was *afraid would happen*.

Sally was able to snap this throwing slump and truly leave her injury behind when she consistently changed her focus of attention. Instead of focusing on the batter—the size of her arms and legs, her batting average and power—all things that scared her, Sally deliberately zeroed in on what had always worked for her—staying loose, trusting herself, and aiming for the catcher's mitt. One way of successfully dealing with your demons is by moving your concentration away from them. Your fears, because they are in the future, are a huge uncontrollable. Dwelling on them will only make you feel more anxious, less confident, and, consequently, more stuck. Refer to our discussion of uncontrollables in Step 2 and developing control over your concentration in Step 3.

Whether it's a fear of failing, making a mistake, getting hurt, or something else, *fear is probably the single biggest cause of choking in sports.* It's a straitjacket that tightens muscles, chokes off breathing, and makes your performance almost unrecognizable. I played some of the sorriest tennis of my competitive career when I was seeded number 1 in a tournament and was preoccupied with fears of losing or embarrassing myself. In game situations where two teams are significantly mismatched, it's not unusual for the underdog to pull off an upset in an unexpectedly close contest when the better team starts playing not to lose.

> *F*ear is probably the single biggest cause
> of choking in sports.

When you play not to lose, your fear makes you too careful. Worrying about the outcome further feeds your fears and makes you play tentatively. Performing tentatively will keep you stuck. Peak performance always comes out of a fearless, go-for-broke attitude. During such a performance, the athletes or team don't think about the outcome. While winning may be critically important to them, it's just not relevant *at the time.* Peak performance requires athletes to go all out at all times. Fear of losing or any other outcome-based fears during a performance can cause athletes to hold back. For example, a pitcher who is afraid of throwing another ball may slow down her arm speed to try to guide the pitch instead of throwing it. The result is often a slow, very hittable pitch.

In 1988 Greg Riddoch was coaching the San Diego Padres, and Tony Gwynn was the team's multimillion-dollar franchise player. Most baseball fans know that Tony is an excellent hitter, and few would ever expect him to be susceptible to a hitting slump. However, in the seven years Riddoch spent coaching him, he saw Gwynn experience one such slump.

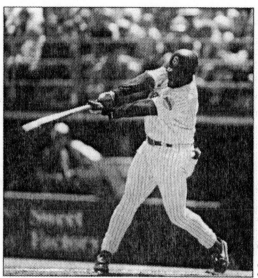

© San Diego Padres/Mike Nowak

At the beginning of 1988, Tony's batting average was about .235. For the first time in his career, he was struggling with hitting. In his mind, he was failing, and his frustration was negatively affecting his attitude.

Two and a half months into the season, the Padres played at Candlestick Park against the San Francisco Giants. It was a cold, windy day and the quiet crowd's energy seemed to be focused on keeping warm rather than cheering. As Riddoch and two other coaches stood outside the dugout and watched, Gwynn stepped up to the plate and hit a pop-up down the right field line. Giants first baseman Will Clark took a few steps and easily caught the ball. What caught Riddoch's attention was that after Gwynn hit the ball, he only ran about halfway to first base, stopped, and then peeled off toward the dugout. He quit running before Clark had even caught the ball. According to Riddoch, this behavior was totally out of character for Tony.

Riddoch told the two coaches he was standing with that he was going to "go get him" and followed Gwynn into the dugout. He sat down next to Tony and said, "You know, T, you have always been a hard-working, never-give-up kind of guy I've encouraged other players to emulate. But I'll be darned if I'm going to use you as an example with the give-up attitude you just showed by not running out that fly. When you act like that, number one, you make me look bad as a manager;

→

and number two, your critics are going to look at you and say that you're not all that great, you can't hit, and you give up before even trying."

Riddoch went on to tell him that he had better not do that again. Gwynn sat there silently, listening attentively to every word his coach said.

After this encounter, Riddoch returned to where the other two coaches were standing outside the dugout. They couldn't wait to hear what he had said to Gwynn. When Riddoch explained that he had basically told Gwynn never to do that again, they were dumbfounded. They warned him that he was "messing with the franchise" and that what he had just done could cost him his job. Riddoch replied, "Let me tell you what my job entails. If I can't say what needs to be said to my players when they aren't showing effort or when they need to be disciplined, then I shouldn't be wearing this uniform. If I lose my job because I'm doing what is right for my players instead of doing what will save my hide, then so be it!" Riddoch simply refused to let his or anyone else's fears interfere with doing exactly what he felt had to be done, no matter what the risks.

The Padres went on to lose that game. After the game, while Riddoch was in the sink area of the coaches' office, Tony approached him. Gwynn calmly set down three crisp $100 bills on the edge of Riddoch's sink, patted him on the back once, and said, "Thanks, Rid—you'll never see that again."

What Riddoch found amazing was that Gwynn had fined himself for behaving out of character. He listened to the hard words his coach had said and used them as a wake-up call on his own. Riddoch's gutsy intervention was apparently exactly what Gwynn had needed. Greg's two colleagues didn't realize that what he had said was actually the right thing. Despite the risk and fear involved in confronting and disciplining a franchise player, what Riddoch did helped him keep his job, not lose it. A successful coach knows his players and pulls no punches because of a player's talent or supposed importance to the team. Riddoch's words helped Gwynn adjust his attitude and he began to work hard again. Within two weeks he had busted out of his hitting slump.

If you're not willing to take risks and move toward your fears as a coach, you won't be successful. Furthermore, if you're closed to outside feedback and unwilling to examine and change your own behaviors, you'll limit yourself as a coach or athlete and be even more vulnerable to performance skids.

This apparent lack of concern for the outcome highlights a paradox in sports and peak performance: To win, when it counts the most, you can't think about winning. To reach your goals, you must let go of them when it's time to compete. Put your commitment, caring, and outcome focus into the long hours of practice, the tough sacrifices, and the day-to-day training. Keeping in mind your goals and dreams *during* practice helps you stay focused and motivated. It will help you keep going when every other part of you is begging to quit. Your goals help you care enough to do what it takes to be successful. However, a goal or outcome focus too close to competition will only feed your performance fears and interfere with staying loose and having fun. We will discuss the proper use of goal setting in more detail in Step 7.

> *T*o beat fear, you must recognize it,
> understand it, and neutralize it.

To beat fear, you must first *recognize* it within yourself, *understand* it, and then *take action* to neutralize it. The rest of this step focuses on these three important elements.

Recognizing Fear

Recognizing fear should not be too difficult. It's a good bet you've been afraid at one time or another in your life. Fear is a universal experience with both positive and negative consequences. In dangerous situations, fear can make you appropriately cautious and lead you to take actions that save your life. In most athletic situations, which aren't inherently life threatening, fear simply short-circuits appropriate responses and causes you to perform poorly.

The experience of fear is a blending of *physiological changes, emotions,* and a special kind of *thinking.* You perceive fear in the environment and feel it in your body as the "fight or flight" response, characterized by faster and more shallow breathing, a rush of adrenaline, tightened muscles, increased heart rate, elevated blood pressure, increased sweating, dry mouth, and cold hands and feet. The emotional experience of fear is felt as anxiety or a sense of unease or dread. Mentally you can recognize that you're afraid because your thoughts start singing the what-ifs and your imagination provides the backup vocals.

The physiological and emotional experience of fear is compelling enough to be impossible to miss. However, the what-ifs within your thoughts may be so habituated by now that you may fail to recognize them for the destructive force that they are. The what-ifs *generate* your fears because they lock your attention on the future and give free reign to your imagination. Under stress, your imagination exaggerates the object of your fear. It takes what you think *could* go wrong, the *possible*, and magnifies it to absurd extremes, the *improbable*. Blowing up fears to the extreme is called "catastrophizing." For example, it's late in the game with the opponent's runners in scoring position. You're at shortstop, catastrophizing. "If I boot the next ball, a run will score, and we'll fall behind. If that happens, we'll probably lose, and it'll be all *my* fault! My error will get me benched and cause the coach to lose confidence in me. I'll probably lose my starting position and, if I don't get to play regularly, I'll lose my edge. Oh, no, if I can't start, no college scouts will get a chance to see me. I won't get that scholarship I've been killing myself for these past six years. Without that scholarship, I won't go to college and my life will be over. . .I'm such a loser. I hope he doesn't hit it to me."

While all these awful occurrences are certainly *possible*, most of them are *not probable*. Entertaining the improbable in this manner *always* generates fear. Furthermore, the future painted by your imagination is a huge uncontrollable. When you focus on uncontrollables, you'll only make yourself more anxious and less confident.

Beating fear starts with an awareness that reciting the what-ifs to yourself will always lead you to the oh, nos ("Oh, no, I choked again!" "Oh, no, another hitless game." "Oh, no, I *did* miss the shot!"). Too many slumping athletes have "inner poets" who recite these fear-inspiring what-ifs to themselves before and during their performances. How would you feel if you regularly listened to your own version of the following poem the night before your big game?

> *As the match approached I began to think*
> *What if I choke? What if I stink?*
> *I could double-fault or land on my head,*
> *What if we lose or my legs feel like lead?*
> *The refs could be blind, missing each call,*
> *What if I drop or bobble the ball?*
> *The beam may be wobbly, the crowd much too big,*
> *What if I get sick or miss a key dig?*
> *My opponent could beat me, I might just get cut,*
> *What if I get hurt or stay stuck in this rut?*
> *The scouts are all here, I could play like a bum,*

What if I strike out and no glory comes?

I know I should relax and just drift off to sleep,

But the what-ifs are endless, all the ways I could weep.

If your inner poet is hard at work scaring you, then silencing him starts with awareness. Are you in the habit of reciting the what-ifs to yourself or anyone else on the team who'll listen? Take a moment to jot down all of your favorites. Get to know them. Fears need a steady diet of what-ifs to grow large and become disruptive. You can begin to starve and then eliminate your fears by *recognizing* and *monitoring* the future-based thinking that feeds them.

Understanding Fear

Once you identify the thinking that fuels fear, you must then come to see it for the terrible liar that it is! While fear is an incredibly powerful emotion within us all, most of the time its facts are either outdated or almost completely fabricated. Fear tricks you into believing things that are not *yet* real. Fear distorts reality with a nonsensical logic that seems to have been borrowed from a five-year-old. It's this childlike logic that then wreaks havoc on you and your performance.

You can begin to eliminate your fears by recognizing and monitoring the future-based thinking that feeds them.

Sports like gymnastics, skating, and diving, where fear of injury is a very real possibility, provide many examples of this childlike logic. A frustrated gymnastics coach recently called me because Andrea, one of his top gymnasts, had "lost" her back handspring on the beam. This skill was relatively basic and one that she had been doing effortlessly for two years. The coach explained that Andrea's back handspring was technically the best in the entire gym. However, no matter what he said or did, he couldn't convince her to execute this skill. Andrea would climb up on the beam with determination etched across her face and then simply freeze. There was absolutely no logical reason for her balking. She had never been injured before, hadn't had any close calls, and had never witnessed another gymnast getting hurt attempting the skill. Intellectually, she knew that she was capable of doing the skill. However, emotionally she was paralyzed. Andrea couldn't even articulate what exactly it was that she feared beyond, "I don't know. I'm just afraid." Her coach's reassurance that she had absolutely nothing to fear had no impact.

Katrina was a former goalkeeper for her country's national soccer team. Before her leg injury she was the starting goalie and played with an aggressiveness and confidence that served her team well. She came out of the goal as necessary, never hesitating to cut off an opponent's shot angle. Her concentration was intense and it enabled her to accurately read the developing play and make some brilliant stops.

In a game two years before I met her, Katrina aggressively came out of the goal to intercept a crossed ball and collided hard with an opponent. The force and angle of the impact broke Katrina's leg in two places and put her out of action for almost a whole year. When she returned to the national team training camp she was a different player. Gone was her daring, aggressive, confident play. She refused to come out of the goal to challenge opponents and especially shied away from crossed balls. Because of her tentative style she was unable to regain her starting position, and her place on the roster seemed to be in jeopardy.

Katrina explained that every time she stepped into the goal she couldn't help but think about her collision and injury. It was as if some bad rerun had gotten stuck in her head and wouldn't shut off. Furthermore, she was quite afraid that she would re-injure herself and so tried to avoid any situation that might result in physical contact. Despite the fact that she was probably the most athletically talented goalkeeper on the team, her fears prevented her from playing that way. This was especially frustrating for her since she was normally aggressive and competitive by nature.

Katrina combined several fear-busting strategies over a six-month period to successfully return her style of play to its old confident and aggressive style. Because her fear wouldn't diminish with refocusing and relaxation strategies, I had Katrina go through the dissociation exercise described in this chapter to help her get distance from her feelings about the accident. Once she was able to do this I encouraged her to spend 15 to 20 minutes a day reviewing past game films that highlighted her old style of play with the instructions to "let your unconscious memorize all the movements and reactions that Katrina displayed." Next I had her gradually move toward her fear by practicing coming out of the goal more and more during scrimmages. This included having her defend against at least 15 cross balls daily in practice games. As she began to feel more comfortable coming out of the goal, her coach gradually increased the physicality of the players she had to stop.

In addition to these strategies, I encouraged Katrina to deal with her fear in the present. That is, every time her mind headed down memory lane, she was instructed to stop those images and instead return her focus to exactly what was happening in the now. Similarly, she practiced exchanging pictures of what she was afraid would happen (another accident) with images of what she wanted to happen (confident, aggressive play). The combination of these strategies helped her put the fear and accident where they belonged, in the past, and soon she was back in the goal for her team.

When a frightened child calls a parent into his room at night because he's *sure* there's a wolf under his bed, showing the child that there's nothing under the bed doesn't always do the trick. Logic will not always comfort a child's raw fear. He *knows* that a wolf is there, despite what anyone says. His terror tells him so. Daddy couldn't see any wolf when he looked because the animal was simply hiding. Many of your performance-related fears, like Andrea's, are as logical as that wolf hiding under the bed. They are the product of your emotions, an active imagination, and distorted knowledge.

> **M**any performance-related fears are the product of your emotions, an active imagination, and distorted knowledge.

The acronym F.E.A.R reflects the idea that fear is really *False Education* that *Appears Real*. On the surface, your fear may seem logical and even warranted. Upon closer examination, however, you'll see that much of this emotion springs from *outdated* and/or *inaccurate* information. For example, a high school springboard diver consistently had trouble with reverse dives. As a senior, she'd been stuck on a reverse-and-a-half for almost a year. Her fear made no sense, given that she would regularly do much more difficult, far scarier dives. When it came to this particular dive, she'd inexplicably freeze. What was *really* stopping her? When we got to the bottom of her problem, we discovered her fear was based on some serious *false education*. When she was nine, she saw her diving idol break her hand on the board attempting this dive. Shocked by this, she reasoned to herself, "If *she's* that good and hurt herself doing the dive, then imagine what will happen to *me* if I try it." Many years later this childhood "learning" and the false logic it was based on conspired to keep her stuck.

Teams that get mired in long losing streaks display a similar false education. For example, a college football team lost 22 games in a row over three seasons. The first year the team was inexperienced and thin on talent, so the consecutive losses were understandable. Despite the addition of a number of talented recruits and transfer students the second year, the team continued its winless ways. After losing the first two games of the third year with an even stronger team, the coach was totally perplexed. His team now had the talent, speed, strength, and experience to win, yet it continued to fall apart whenever victory was near. It was as if the losing streak had taken on a life of its own.

The real problem lay in the minds of the athletes and the collective consciousness of the team. Mentally, they played like the team of the past that started the losing streak. The team *expected* to lose because that was something they *always* did. Despite the fact that this information was now outdated, the players unknowingly looked for *signs* during the game that "it" was beginning to happen again—for example, a drive-ending fumble, a dropped touchdown pass, a great score by the opponent, or a momentum-stopping penalty. The players then used these "signs" to convince themselves that another failure was close at hand. The familiar signs of disaster would then trigger feelings of hopelessness and giving up.

When you're stuck in a slump, you view your world through the lenses of failure. You "see" numerous opportunities for repeating the unhappy past everywhere you look. You harbor the expectation that it is impossible to succeed. You tend to misread competitive situations to support this negative view and scare yourself. The normal bad breaks, setbacks, or poor calls during competition are misinterpreted as signs that you're about to self-destruct *again*.

Are your fears based on this kind of false education? A tennis pro once told me that whenever he was ahead 5 games to 2 in the deciding set, he'd always lose! How did he "learn" this? Over the past two years he had lost several key matches after being that close to victory. He used this false information to feed his negative beliefs and to hunt down additional signs that "it" was going to happen again. The fear of failure that he found every time further contributed to his inability to close out his matches.

Athletes frequently use this kind of false education to fuel their fears and sabotage their performance. Superstitions are closely related to fear. A superstition is an *illogical* belief that links *how* you perform with seemingly unrelated events or behaviors. Athletes are often a superstitious lot who look for external explanations for their successes and failures. Superstitious thoughts like, "This field is jinxed. . .we can never win here," "I've got my lucky socks on," "I have to eat spaghetti the night before I race or else," or "Unless I get to do my special ritual, things will go terribly wrong" have almost no basis in reality. However, this kind of thinking provides "signs" that *convince* the athlete that something good or bad is going to happen, and *because* of these thoughts, it usually does.

Sam, a college baseball player, demonstrates the irrational power of superstitions and how this kind of thinking combines with fear to fuel slumps. Sam believed that whenever a plane flew overhead while he was batting, it would cause him to strike out. Unfortunately for him, his home field was near a large metropolitan airport and directly under the approach to its main runway. Instead of relaxing at the plate and concentrating on the ball and the pitcher's release point, Sam diverted some of his attention to nervously scanning the skies with his eyes and ears for approaching aircraft. His "fear" of airplanes fed his fear of striking out and caused his hitting to slump.

Tony, a 16-year-old wrestler, demonstrates the positive effect that superstitions can have on your performance. Tony believed that for him to wrestle well in competition, he had to go through a very specific ritual. First, he'd close his eyes and see an image of his smiling 6-year-old brother hugging him and saying, "You can do it, Tony. I know you can do it! Do it for me." Next he'd take his warm-up pants off, removing his left leg before the right. He then would follow the same order taking off his jacket. When he stretched he always worked on the left side of his body before the right. Similarly, he had a set pattern of warm-up exercises that he *always* did before the match. By the time he walked onto the mat, he felt confident and ready. His superstitious ritual kept him calm and focused, regardless of who he was wrestling or how big the match.

Both superstition and fear spring from illogical, childlike reasoning. This reasoning reflects the "learning by association" process of very young children. If a six-year-old breaks a dish in the dining room and hears her parents fighting in the basement, she immediately thinks that *she* caused the fight by breaking the dish. Similarly, when Wade Boggs played for the Boston Red Sox and went 3 for 4 one night after eating a chicken dinner, he associated his success with that pregame meal. Chicken then became his dinner of choice on game day. The hockey player who spits on his stick before he goes on the ice developed this superstitious ritual in a similar way. On a night that he happened to do this for the first time, he had two assists and scored two goals. He then began to *associate* his good play and points earned with the spitting. Presto! A superstition is born.

Are irrational beliefs contributing to your slump? Like Tony's, rituals and superstitions can be a positive, calming force as long as you can *control* them. If your rituals or superstitions involve circumstances beyond your control, they will end up controlling you. For example, a placekicker on a high school football team needed *all* his teammates to touch his kicking foot before he went out for a field goal. In his mind, this ritual appeased the kicking gods and guaranteed that they would carry his ball straight and far, directly through the uprights. In one of their bigger and rougher games of the season, he was called onto the field with 15 seconds remaining to erase a two point deficit and win the game. As he lined up his teammates on the sidelines for their ritual touch, he nervously realized that two key players were missing. They had been injured earlier and taken from the field to a nearby hospital. As he walked onto the field, he was feeling a sense of dread. He was *afraid* that without his missing teammates' "magic touch," he'd miss the kick. Because that was all he focused on when he went out for the kick, he was right!

When facing a superstition that's working against you, understand that you, not the superstition, have control.

When developing effective team and individual rituals, be sure they do not involve uncontrollables. It's the uncontrollable aspect of superstitions that gets athletes into trouble and fuels their fears. As I mentioned in the previous step's discussion of preperformance rituals, keep your rituals short and simple. When facing a superstition that's working against you, understand that *you*, not the superstition, have the real control. If for some reason you can't do what your ritual or superstition demands, stay calm. Not doing the ritual won't hurt you. What will hurt you is what you say to yourself and focus on as a result of this break in your routine. To help you control your superstitions, refer to the following fear-busting strategies, particularly the discussions on changing the focus of concentration and challenging the fear's logic.

Defeating Fear

The last step in mastering your fears is to take action in dealing with them. When confronted with fear, most people become overwhelmed and use the F.E.A.R. strategy they learned in childhood: *Forget Everything And Run.* Fear is a rather unpleasant emotion, and most of us have been programmed to skillfully avoid it. You don't raise your hand to answer the question. You leave the double-back out of your gymnastics routine. You stop doing the double axel. You hope that the ball isn't hit to you. You don't volunteer to go out and take that penalty kick in the shoot-out. You stop playing aggressively. You simply refuse to get back up on the proverbial horse after it dumped you. To defeat your fears, however, you must learn to move toward rather than away from them, using the following strategies.

Move Toward the Fear

A funny thing happens when you move *toward* instead of *away from* your fears. They begin to change right before your eyes. They get smaller and lose their power. In a paradoxical way, allowing yourself to get close to and examine your fears, to face them squarely, is what helps you neutralize them. Fear can only have power over you if you continually avoid it. Your avoidance of a fearful situation is what enables the fear to grow. Avoiding fear allows your imagination to continue to contribute to the "false education" that supports the emotion. It's only by moving toward your fears that you can see the fallacies behind them.

Dr. Rob Gilbert, a sport psychologist, once asked legendary boxing trainer

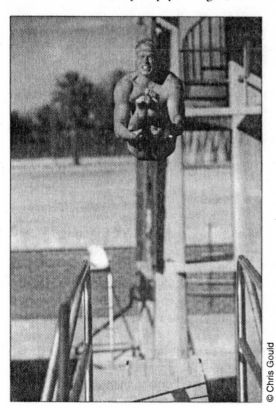

© Chris Gould

Teddy Atlas how he taught his athletes to overcome the fear that was so much a part of boxing. Atlas, who had worked with a number of boxing greats, including Mike Tyson, explained that boxing is very much like war. In war there are two kinds of soldiers, the hero and the coward. According to Atlas, the major difference between a hero and a coward is not fear. Both the hero and the coward feel fear. The key difference lies in how each deals with the feeling. The hero feels his fear and moves toward it, doing the fearful thing anyway. The coward feels the fear and moves away from the fear-generating situation.

*Fear can only have power over you
if you continually avoid it.*

What Atlas said is very basic to defeating those demons that may be haunting you. To beat fear, you must force yourself to get up and do the thing that you're most afraid of, over and over again. If you are afraid to face a really fast pitcher, execute a double axel, do a reverse-and-a-half, or perform a back handspring, then you need to put yourself in these situations again and again. You need to find the fastest pitchers to practice hitting against, try to set a record for the most double axels ever attempted in one practice session, do literally hundreds of the reverse-and-a-half dives, or attempt as many back handsprings as possible. Taking action in this way loosens the grip that fear has on you, because it is difficult to fear the familiar. Fear's power lies in its unfamiliarity. The avoidance inherent in fear keeps you from getting comfortable and familiar. Familiarity dissipates anxiety. It's the unknown that holds the terror.

Break Up the Fear

The riddle "How do you eat an elephant?" has a simple answer that can help you systematically disarm your fears—"one bite at a time." If you try to swallow an entire limb at once, you'll develop a crushing stomachache. Performance fears are like that elephant. You need to tackle them in small pieces.

You need to tackle performance fears in small pieces.

This is certainly not a new idea for athletes. "Chunking down" an obstacle or technique into its component parts and then attacking these parts one at a time will enable you to do the seemingly impossible. A diver learns a scary new reverse by "chunking down" the dive into its "lead-up" skills. Working on all the lead-up skills enables the entire dive to come together. This is the "divide and conquer" strategy. You attack that fear a little bit at a time.

Let's say you're terrified to play in front of huge crowds or against certain opponents. You can begin to chunk that fear down by mentally practicing being successful in front of that crowd or opponent. In the safety of your room, you mentally see, hear, and feel yourself playing comfortably and confidently. You "experience" yourself performing exactly the way you'd like to, completely unfazed by those uncontrollables. Your imagery practice becomes the first bite of the elephant. We will further discuss the use

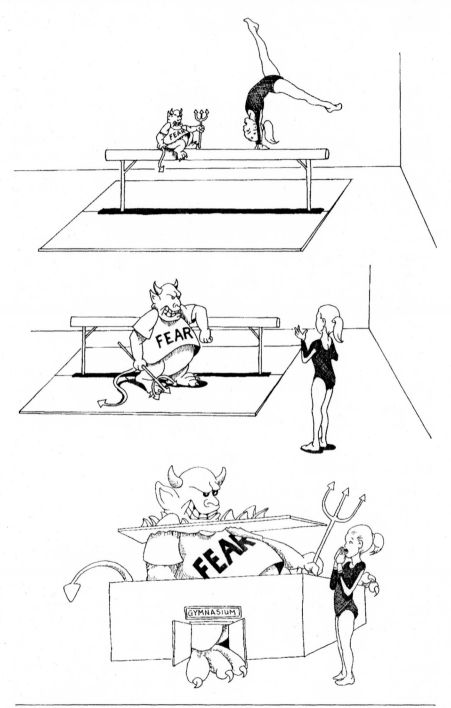

Avoidance feeds fear.

of mental rehearsal in Step 6. Additional "bites" include practicing with progressively larger audiences or scrimmaging against tougher and tougher opponents.

I used this chunking-down strategy to help Sally, the eighth-grade softball pitcher we discussed previously in this step, beat her fear. After having been hit in the face by a line drive, Sally was much too frightened to actually practice against hard hitters. She was, however, able to mentally rehearse throwing against them while still feeling calm and confident. Once she was quite comfortable with this "practice," we had her start pitching against older players who she knew were weak hitters. In the next step we included slightly better hitters in the lineup. When Sally was able to maintain her confidence and composure, we added even stronger hitters until she was no longer distracted by the batter or the past.

Coaches teaching scary skills naturally use this "eat-an-elephant" strategy. They break down the difficult skills into "small bites" and teach these one at a time. Working in this way slowly "desensitizes" the athlete to the fear and helps her master the new move. This is the coaching technique of helping your athletes *get comfortable being uncomfortable.* By gradually and continually putting the athlete into an uncomfortable situation, moving toward the fear, you will help the athlete ultimately become comfortable with it.

For example, in a fly-away, the gymnast swings forward, completely stretched out, back parallel to the floor, and then releases the bar, does a back flip, and lands to end the routine. A gymnast who is afraid to perform a fly-away could first get comfortable with the process of swinging and letting go by just practicing this part of the skill into a pile of mats or a "pit." Next, the coach could have the gymnast do the entire move while hooked to a harness. Finally, the gymnast could do the fly-away with the coach providing a hand spot.

Reframe the Fear

When Beth qualified for her first nationals, she was absolutely ecstatic for the three weeks preceding the meet. However, at the meet site she began to consider the reality of the situation. She was about to compete against some of the best swimmers in the country, and she was starting to feel intimidated. Beth couldn't believe that she was actually on the same deck with some of the athletes she had been reading about in her swim magazine. Swim against them! All she could think about was getting their autographs!

Frank was a striker on a select soccer team. He was just coming back from missing several months of play after severely spraining his ankle.

Though the doctor had finally cleared him to play again, he felt like a different player. He lacked the aggressiveness and confidence that used to be so much a part of his game. He felt tentative and preoccupied with fears that he would re-injure himself.

In these two scenarios the athletes' fears are confidence-eroding. The athletes are confronted with situations outside of their comfort zones. When you move up to a higher level of competition or return after a serious injury, you feel stretched to your limits physically and mentally. Fear is a *natural* response to this kind of challenge. However, when you *misread* these fears (with thoughts like "I don't belong here," "We're going to get totally embarrassed," and "What if I sprain that ankle again?"), you'll end up distracted and intimidated. Reframing or *changing the meaning of the fear in a positive way* will help you get beyond it.

F*ear is the gateway to improvement.*

What does fear *really* mean in these situations? It's the gateway to improvement. You have to pass through the fear to get to the next level. Feeling fear means that you're "pushing the envelope." Playing out of your league the first few times is supposed to be scary. Keeping this in mind will take away some of the fear's power. Even in the case of an injury, the fear that you feel as you attempt to return to top form is a natural and positive marker that lets you know that you're on the right track. Experiencing the fear of re-injury is actually the last step in the total rehabilitation process, before the injury is completely forgotten.

Change the Focus of Concentration

Earlier in this step I mentioned that fear is a product of the what-ifs. When your concentration leaves the *now* of the performance and jumps ahead to the *future*, which is an uncontrollable, the result will almost always be fear. (Refer to Step 2 for an in-depth discussion of uncontrollables and to Step 3 for more details on the here-and-now rule for peak performance.) One of your most important fear-busting strategies is to keep yourself mentally focused on what you can control before and during the performance. Monitor your focus of concentration whenever you're in a potentially fearful situation, so that you stay in the now. It's critical that you don't allow the what-ifs any airtime in your head. When you become aware that you're starting to listen to this fear-inspiring poetry (*What if I get beat, What if my opponent starts to cheat*), you need to quickly bring your attention back to the things you can control.

*K*eep yourself mentally focused on what you can control
before and during the performance.

For example, I once worked with a college hammer thrower who got great distance in practice but always seemed to find a way to mess up in the bigger meets. She had been struggling for well over a year with this problem, which we traced to a fear of embarrassment. The previous year at a dual meet, she lost her balance in the middle of a throw and fell on her face. It was her fear of embarrassment more than anything else that seemed to plague her from then on. When she was able to switch her focus away from the what-ifs to the elements that helped her throw well, she began to improve and consistently throw her best under pressure.

Challenge the Fear's Logic

One way of working through your fears is to confront the childlike logic and catastrophizing that forms its foundation. Rather than listening to the self-talk of your inner coach telling you it's the end of the world, begin to question and even refute the arguments your inner coach generates. If that inner voice is scaring you, don't sit back and listen. Yes, you struck out your last six at-bats, but this is a *new* one and anything can happen *now* so

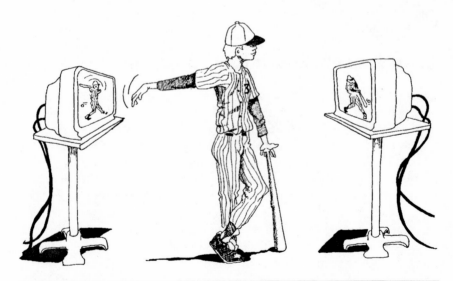

Change your focus.

keep your focus. Besides, didn't you go 8 for 10 four weeks ago? Sure, you're worried about "dying" in the middle of the race, but you're in great physical shape, have never died before, and can easily run six 440s in a row in practice. Or, you may agree that you are afraid about what others will say if you lose, but what's the worst that could happen? And so what if the coach benches you? You'll just work harder until you regain your starting position. And there's no way they'll throw you off the team if you mess up. Everyone makes mistakes!

When it's appropriate (don't do this in the middle of your performance, when your focus should be in the competition), dispute the catastrophic and mostly nonsensical reasoning behind your fears. With a little practice, your arguments will help loosen the grip that your fears have on you and rebuild your shaky confidence. These counter-arguments will seem phony and difficult to believe at first. This is expected, especially if you're talented and practiced at scaring yourself. Be persistent and don't allow yourself to give in to the fears. Remember, *you can talk yourself into and out of anything.*

> **C**onfront the childlike logic and catastrophizing that forms the foundation of fear.

A good way to talk yourself out of your fears is to become your own "best coach." When you're struggling and scared, what would a really good coach say to you? How would this ideal coach deal with your fears? What would he or she say when you failed? Take over the dialogue and perspective of this ideal coach.

Create Distance From the Fear

Several years ago I worked with a 17-year-old springboard diver who was terrified of doing reverse dives. Whenever she was forced to execute this dive she'd either freeze or jump the dive out too far from the board. Proper execution of this dive requires the athlete to "take the dive up" over the board. Despite an incapacitating fear, Johanna was still one of the better divers in her state. However, her block on reverses dramatically limited her potential.

When Johanna was 12 and just learning a reverse somersault, she accidentally hit her feet on the board during an entry, and the force of the blow stripped several toenails from her feet. Five years later that accident and the fear it engendered continued to paralyze her. Emotionally, Johanna acted as if the accident had just happened. Her coach had tried to get her to move toward her fear and chunk it down into small pieces. He told her that it was normal to be afraid and that every diver has to go through fear to get better. He had her switch her focus of concentration away from what she was afraid would happen to elements in the dive. He even tried to get her to argue with the fear's logic. But no matter what they tried together, nothing could loosen the powerful grip that the fear held on Johanna.

If trying to shake a performance fear leaves you feeling like you're trying to outrun your own shadow, despair not! The reason may be that you're simply "too close" to the memory of that fear-inspiring incident. This is exactly why Johanna had been unable to get free from her fear, even though the accident happened five years ago. Every time she thought of doing a reverse dive, she would remember her accident by *associating* or stepping back *inside* the memory, reliving everything that had happened.

Most people remember things by having *dissociated* images or pictures. That is, you see yourself performing from a distance, from the sports fan's perspective. This keeps you free from the powerful feelings attached to the original experience. By associating, you relive the experience, which is why, years later, it can remain as powerful as the day it happened. Individuals who suffer from post-traumatic stress disorder, such as war veterans and accident victims, have flashbacks that seem real, because they step back inside their memories and relive the terrible emotions again and again.

> **T**o get distance from a persistent fear, you have to separate your feelings from the visual images in your memory.

When everything you've tried has failed and your fear continues to immobilize you, your next step is to create distance for yourself. To get distance from a really persistent fear, you have to dissociate or separate your feelings from the visual images in your memory. Once you do this, your fear will lose power over you. The following exercise, taken from neurolinguistic programming, will teach you this dissociation or distancing process.[3] You may need to practice it several times to help you neutralize those strong feelings.

CREATING DISTANCE

Imagine that you're sitting in the middle of a movie theater, and on the screen you see a black-and-white snapshot of yourself in the original fear-inducing situation. This snapshot shows the situation just before things went bad.

Now, imagine that you can float out of your body up to the projection booth in the theater where you can watch yourself watching yourself. From that position, you'll be able to see yourself sitting in the middle of the theater and also see yourself in the still frame on the screen.

Next, imagine you can turn that snapshot into a black-and-white movie, and, *staying mentally in the projection booth*, watch it from the beginning to just beyond the end of the unpleasant experience. It is critical here that you watch yourself watching yourself while the movie plays, *seeing and hearing only* what is going on in the movie, feeling no emotions.

Finally, when you get to the end of the movie, freeze the last frame as a slide. Then imagine that you can leave the projection booth, jump down into the theater, and then jump up on the screen. Imagine that you can jump inside that final frame, and then run the movie *backward*. All the people will walk backward and everything will happen in reverse, just as if you were rewinding a movie, except you'll be *inside* the movie. Run it backward *in color*, taking about two seconds to do the whole film.

I first asked Johanna to indicate, by distance away from her body, how closely she was still experiencing her diving injury (that is, a foot away would indicate that the incident feels like it just happened today; ten feet, last week; thirty feet, last month; and so on). She put this five-year-old accident right in front of her! After we did this dissociation exercise the first time, she was able to move the mishap forty feet away. Continued practice helped Johanna get some much-needed emotional distance, and soon she was freed up enough to start doing reverse dives again.

Conclusion

Remember, if fear is at work within your slump, don't listen to its deceitful "words of wisdom." Fear is a skilled liar that deftly twists the truth and victimizes your confidence. If you let your fears run the show, you'll stop believing in yourself. When fear undercuts your all-important belief in yourself, performance problems will soon follow. Furthermore, fear prevents you from creating positive images in your mind's eye. Fear tricks you into believing that your goals aren't achievable and that mental toughness is not something you can feel. Take action. Move toward and challenge your fears. You have more power than you think.

As you face your fears, you'll recapture a sense of personal power. Perhaps you'll even notice that your "slump attitude" is beginning to improve. Facing and moving toward your fears will also help you restart old familiar feelings of personal control. That is, you'll start to believe in yourself again. As your confidence and belief in yourself increase, you'll begin to regularly "see what you want to happen" during performances. Your ability to create these positive images will further loosen the slump's grip on you, help you begin to set big goals again, and further contribute to mental toughness.

In the next step in our slump-busting model, "Expecting Success," you'll learn how to develop and enhance this all-important belief in yourself. As an athlete, you're limited by what you believe is possible. Much of athletic performance is self-fulfilling—that is, you usually get what you expect. "Expecting Success" will show you how to do just that—expect success.

5

EXPECTING
SUCCESS

"If you think you are beaten, you are;
If you think that you dare not, you don't;
If you'd like to win, but you think you can't,
it's almost certain you won't."

As I discussed in Step 4, fear closes the door on peak performance and locks you into a slump. I presented some techniques that you can use to neutralize some of the paralyzing effects of fear, especially when that fear is related to physical injury, such as getting hit by a ball, hitting the diving board, or missing a release move in gymnastics. However, fears are more often related to mental wounds than physical—fear of failing, making mistakes, or letting the team down—and therefore require different strategies to overcome. A primary strategy for attacking mental fears is learning to control your focus of concentration (discussed in detail in Step 3). Additional fear-busting techniques are woven through later steps in the model—mental rehearsal in Step 6, goal setting in Step 7, boosting self-confidence in Step 8, reframing and mastering failures in Step 9, and handling competitive pressures in Step 10.

In this step we will zero in on one primary source of these mental-based fears, your beliefs, and teach you how to turn them around so that they work *for* rather than *against* you. If you don't really believe in yourself, then you'll enter competition entertaining the what-ifs and expecting failure.

Unfortunately, these worries and negative expectations shape your performance. To bust that slump, you must learn to expect success and to believe in yourself. You must challenge those negative, slump-fueling beliefs that have forced their way into your consciousness. As an athlete, you are limited *most* by what you *believe* is possible. Belief is a key ingredient in peak performance. When you believe in yourself, there are few limits to how high you can fly. However, if you doubt yourself, you'll never even get off the ground. To get yourself airborne again, you must learn to expect success.

*Y*ou are limited most by what you believe is possible.

For example, several months ago a talented distance swimmer telephoned me and complained about her inability to make her Junior National cuts in the mile. She had been struggling with this time block for nearly a year and couldn't understand why she kept missing it. What was especially frustrating to Jamie was that she had easily broken the cut by 13 seconds in practice on a day when she was already quite tired. However, in meets she'd become too preoccupied with her past failures, how awful she felt, and whether or not she'd flop in the middle *again*. The harder Jamie tried, the worse she seemed to do. She was feeling discouraged and completely hopeless. Like every slumping athlete, Jamie had stopped *believing* in herself and had begun to expect failure. Her lack of belief contributed to her poor performances under pressure and kept her stuck.

The Power of Belief

Belief can help you find the possible in every impossible. It can take ordinary ability and elevate it to the extraordinary. It's that unknown catalyst that, when added to the equation, makes everything wonderfully unpredictable. It transforms the whole into something more than its component parts. For example, in 1990, heavyweight world champion boxer Mike Tyson stepped into the ring to defend his title against James "Buster" Douglas, a perennial loser with a reputation for quitting. The fight was so mismatched that the bookies weren't even taking bets on the outcome. Everyone *knew* that Tyson was going to win. The only interesting question on everyone's mind was what minute of the fight would Douglas hit the canvas.

But Buster Douglas was on a personal mission and had a hidden advantage. He alone *believed* that he had a chance to beat Tyson. It didn't matter that everyone else saw Tyson as unstoppable and viewed this bout as the mismatch of the century. Douglas had dedicated the fight to his recently deceased mother and believed in his heart that she was in his corner. His belief helped him rock Tyson and the entire fight world as he pulled off one of the greatest upsets in boxing history, twice knocking Tyson down and scoring a TKO.

How many times in sports do we witness the incredible power of belief in propelling athletes and teams to accomplish the seemingly impossible? Unseeded and unknown American runner Billy Mills came from 10 meters back to beat defending world champion Ron Clark to win the 10,000-meter run at the 1964 Tokyo Olympics. The amazing Mets of 1969 came out of nowhere to win the World Series. In the 1980 "miracle on ice," the U.S. hockey team upset the invincible Soviet team on its way to winning Olympic gold. Duke University upset the unbeaten defending champion UNLV Running Rebels to win the 1991 NCAA basketball championship. In these and every other athletic upset, the victors have a powerful self-belief sitting on their bench.

Success and Failure Cycles

A positive belief always propels you toward success. If you expect to win, you treat failures, obstacles, and injuries differently than if you expect failure. When the going gets bumpy, you simply become more tenacious. You refuse to quit. Setbacks further fuel your motivation and determination to succeed. Your positive belief sets up a "self-fulfilling prophecy" in which you end up getting what you expect. Because you *believe* you can, you *do*. Furthermore, the success that you finally earn confirms and strengthens your original positive beliefs. Thus, a success cycle is set into motion. Because you *believe* you can, you *do*; and because you *do*, you *believe* you can.

Athletes in the middle of a winning streak demonstrate a simple, positive relationship:

Positive Expectations ⟶ Success ⟶ Positive Expectations

You see a similar self-fulfilling prophecy at work with slumping athletes, only it operates in reverse. Athletes in the middle of a losing streak or slump demonstrate a negative relationship:

Negative Expectations ⟶ Failure ⟶ Negative Expectations

Because struggling athletes do not believe in themselves and expect to fail, their view of setbacks and obstacles merely reinforces their negativity. When things go wrong, they think, "I knew this was going to happen" or "Here we go again." Because they expect failure, they have little determination to succeed in the face of these obstacles. Setbacks and failures sap their motivation, and their efforts in battling back are half-hearted. Consequently, they fail again, reconfirming their original belief of "I can't." A negative failure cycle is set into motion and maintains the slump. Because you *believe* you can't, you *don't*; and because you *don't*, you *believe* you can't.

The self-fulfilling cycle that operates in winning and losing streaks is diagrammed in figure 5.1 When you're "on" as an athlete, your successes generate positive, affirming self-talk. Because of this inner dialogue, your self-confidence is enhanced and feeds a positive belief in yourself and your abilities. The resulting expectation of success keeps you calm, confident, and composed as you go into your next performance. These feelings allow you to easily maintain the right focus of concentration so critical to performing to your potential. Another good performance simply reinforces the positive self-talk, starting the cycle over again.

In a losing streak or slump, the cycle is negative rather than positive. In Jamie's slump, for example, failure to make her Junior National cut generates negative self-talk, like "You're so slow," "I can't believe you blew it again," and "Everyone else is qualifying, what's wrong with *you?*" As a result of this self-inflicted emotional beating, Jamie has even more self-doubts and less confidence. These feelings, in turn, lead to her negative beliefs about the next time she tries to qualify: "I wonder if I'll *ever* make my cuts. I'm really not sure that I will." Jamie now expects to fail. Her negative beliefs and expectations of failure ("I hope I don't die. What if it happens again?") generate anxiety, which tightens her muscles and interferes with maintaining the concentration necessary to go fast. As a result, when she races, her focus is in her head instead of in the experience. Consequently, she swims poorly, which triggers more negative self-talk, and the cycle repeats itself, reinforcing her failures.

If you can *begin to believe* in yourself again, this slump cycle can be turned around. To do this, you must first attack and weaken those already existing negative beliefs. For example, I started an assault on Jamie's negative self-beliefs right after she finished presenting her problem to me. I indirectly challenged her belief that she'd never qualify and got her to consider the possibility of success by asking, "I wonder if you'll be surprised at how quickly *you're going to get over this block?* Sooner or later most athletes I work with are wonderfully puzzled at how short a time it actually takes them to get unstuck."

This question and statement confused her and put her in a double bind. To answer yes or no to the question, she had to assume that she was going to quickly bust the slump. Her answer didn't change the implication hidden within the question and statement of fast relief from her performance woes.

The Cycle of Success

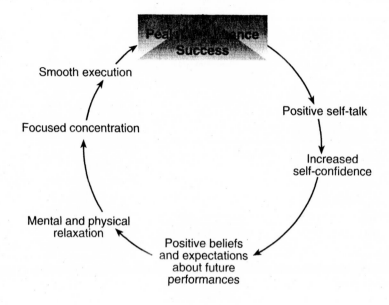

The Cycle of Failure

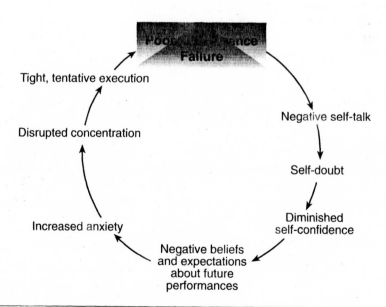

Figure 5.1 The success and failure cycles.

How do you begin to expect success when failure always seems to be knocking at your door? How do you turn your failure-fueled beliefs around when you can't see anything to be positive about? Can you even *remember* what it was like to feel self-confident and believe in yourself? It seems relatively easy to expect success when things are always going your way. How you do this when you're struggling is another story entirely. If you're stuck in a slump, these questions just don't seem to have adequate answers.

> **I**f you can begin to believe in yourself again,
> the slump cycle can be turned around.

When you're struggling, it's as if your best performances are held captive by the slump behind a huge fortress of negative beliefs. These negative beliefs wall off your great performances and leave you with only memories of failure. Your slump is both maintained and protected by these steep walls. Peak performance can only happen if you're able to break them down. As an athlete, you may have been attacking these walls for months. All your attempts to crash through these walls have been repelled ("I've changed my grip, stance, timing, strategy, technique, diet, dress, and even my hair style, yet *nothing* has helped."). You are tired and impatient ("I can't believe this is *still* going on. No one else is struggling like me. *Everybody else* in the gym can do this skill! Enough already!"). You're frustrated and confused ("I have no idea what else I can do to try to stop this.") and your morale is low ("I'll never get that scholarship now."). You have even considered giving up ("Why bother anymore. I might as well just quit."). You have to do something *now*. How can you effectively bust through those walls and release your peak performance?

The Structure of Belief

When planning your assault against the slump, you need to know as much about the enemy as possible. What are your negative beliefs? How are they constructed? What feeds them? Do they have any weaknesses? What weapons will be most effective in removing them? Are any of these available to you now?

If self-limiting belief is the enemy, what do we know about it? First, we know that *belief* is a *conviction* that certain things are *true*. It's a *mental acceptance* of this truth, even though evidence doesn't support *absolute certainty*. For example, a soccer coach got his team to believe that they *always* played better whenever the weather and field conditions were terrible. In the beginning of the season, he renamed his team "Mickey's Mudders" to reflect the belief he wanted to cultivate. When the skies opened up and the field turned to mud, their play *always* shone. He was tired of listening to complaints like "We need better field conditions to play *our* game," "We can't play in the mud," and "When the field is slippery, we always lose." He knew that his team's negative beliefs adversely affected its play in these situations.

There was little, if any, absolute truth in what coach Mickey was saying. The *truth* lay in how his players performed once they bought the belief that he was selling. While they played great under sunny skies, *believing* they played even better in the rain kept them calm and confident whenever the weather turned foul. As Mickey told me, "At first it didn't matter if it was *really* true that they played better in the mud. All that mattered was that they all *believed* it. Once they believed it, they actually began to play better."

To break down the walls of self-limiting beliefs and replace them with performance-enhancing ones, it would be useful to know how that wall is put together. As illustrated in figure 5.2, beliefs have their base in the *experiences* that you have in and out of sports. But it's not the experiences per se that are important as much as the *self-talk about these experiences*. It's not how you play, what mistakes you make, or what the fans yell at you that shape your beliefs, but how you *interpret* these things to yourself. Beliefs really get their start with your self-talk. Finally, your beliefs impel you to *action*.

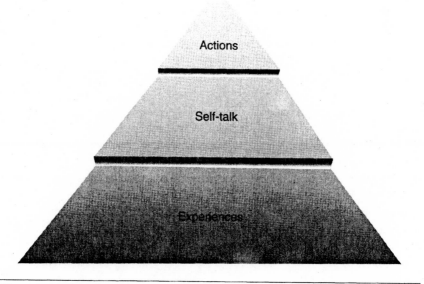

Figure 5.2 The structure of belief.

The Red Devils high school baseball team seemed to have losing down to an exact science after dropping 12 straight games at the end of last season and 9 in a row to start this season. To make matters more frustrating for the coaches and players, many of these losses were by just a few runs. Of the 21 losses, only 5 were downright blowouts. It wasn't like the Red Devils were bad players, either. They had their share of talent both in the field and at the plate. It was just that when the game was on the line, their bats got quiet and their defense fell apart.

By the fifth game this year, the team as a whole expected to lose. Even when they were in control of a game, not too far from everyone's consciousness was the very real fear that they would probably find a way to snatch defeat from the jaws of victory. And so far their negative expectations had been uncannily accurate. Expecting something terrible to happen, the Devils would start playing tentatively and soon their control and lead would evaporate. "Oh no, here we go again, this *always* happens" became like a twisted mantra for the team. The Red Devils wonderfully demonstrated the repetitive and self-maintaining cycle of a losing streak—one loss begets another, which begets another, and so on.

After talking with the staff I met with the team and focused my comments on helping them get back in control. I wanted them to understand that their negative thinking and expectations were the primary culprits in maintaining their slump. The message was very simple: "If you want to bust that slump, you have to start believing in yourselves again and expecting to win." To help them do this we developed some team rules about their negativity and overuse of "permanent language" comments like "We *always* lose" and "We can *never* win the close ones." Because of its "garbage in, garbage out" impact, negativity was outlawed for the rest of the season. Players immediately began policing themselves the next day, quickly reminding each other whenever anything negative popped out in practice.

Next all the players made a commitment to leave the past in the past, because those 21 games were behind them and nothing could be done to change that. They committed to approach each game in the now, playing one inning at a time. Picking up on the comment that the now is the only time zone that you can play good ball in, the team captain suddenly jumped up in the middle of the workshop and asked his teammates if they knew what time it was. As a group, the players yelled out, "It's now!" whereupon the captain responded like a drill sergeant, "I can't hear you. What time is it?" The team yelled "Now!" even louder and a new pre- and during-game focusing ritual was started.

Several players took some of the ideas they had heard in the workshop, and positive affirmation signs appeared on the locker room walls the next day. The statements included "It's NOW until the final out," "Positive Is Power," and "If you think you can or think you can't, you're right...and Red Devils CAN!" The Devils took to heart the "acting as if" strategy and everyone on the team made a deliberate effort to keep his physical posture up and to smile no matter what was going on in the game.

Their new attitude served them well in their next game. They quickly jumped out to a 4–0 lead and maintained the scoring advantage until their opponents' last at-bat. With two outs and a pitch away from snapping their losing streak, the Devils watched in horror as a rally tied the game and sent it into extra innings. The old Devils would have crumbled and folded at this point. The new, more positive Devils got even more focused and determined. The coach told me the dugout was bursting with intense, positive chatter at that point. This only increased when their opponents put a runner in scoring position with one out. Undaunted, the defense made an incredible double play to end the threat. The team was so pumped when they got back to the dugout that the coach knew the opposing pitcher was in serious trouble. Forgotten were the 21 losses in a row and expectations of failure. The Devils *knew* they were going to win the game in their half of the inning. Two singles and a double later, the Devils won the game and officially snapped out of their slump.

For example, you have an experience of overhearing a respected coach talking about you to an assistant: "Y'know, I'm really impressed with Kelly. She's a great leader, really handles pressure well, and has a good head on her shoulders. I think she has tremendous potential and is really going to make a huge contribution to our team this year." Perhaps you didn't really believe this about yourself, but having this *experience* of accidentally eavesdropping on the coach sets off a certain line of thinking. Maybe when you go out for practice that day, you can't get the coach's words out of your head. Replaying them over and over shapes your *self-talk*. You start to see yourself just a bit the way the coach was describing. You begin to feel better about yourself and more confident. You start *acting* differently. When you are in a situation that demands leadership, you hear the coach's words in your head and surprise yourself by taking charge. A belief has been planted and is taking root.

Olympic backstroker (1992, 1996) Trippi Schwenk was 7 years old when he first started swimming. At his first end-of-the-year banquet, the club hosted Kim Linnehan, a former Olympian, as the keynote speaker. Kim looked out over the two hundred young, attentive faces and said, "You never know what you can achieve in this sport and in life. You never know how far you can go when you set your mind to something. In fact, one or two of you listening to me tonight will probably even go on to make it to the Olympics." Young Schwenk heard those words and *thought* the Olympian was talking directly to *him*. To an impressionable kid, that experience became the basis of a dream that shaped his life. It generated a certain kind of self-talk that began to form the foundation for his beliefs.

Your beliefs begin to emerge out of your self-talk. Perhaps this is where the saying "you become what you think about most of the time" comes from. Certainly the thoughts that bounce around in your head shape what you believe. Since your beliefs then influence behavior, they set a self-fulfilling prophecy or cycle in motion. Your inner dialogue also triggers the formation of emotion, which attaches itself to your belief and further affects performance. For example, negative self-talk creates negative feelings. If you tell yourself you're a head case who *always* chokes under pressure, you'll feel depressed, discouraged, and incompetent.

Breaking Down Negative Beliefs

As we've discussed, the main building blocks of beliefs are *experience* and *self-talk* (see figure 5.2). Your beliefs then impel you to *action*. You can break down beliefs by attacking any of these elements: experience, self-talk, or action. While negative beliefs sometimes seem etched in stone, they *can* be changed. With the right kind of assault in just the right places, you can break down the building blocks of the negative beliefs and replace them with positive ones.

Y*ou can break down beliefs by attacking any of these elements: experience, self-talk, or action.*

So beginning with the foundation and progressing up the pyramid of your belief structure, let's assault your negative beliefs so you can get your performances back on track. Starting with changing your experience, then your self-talk, and finally your actions, here are some techniques you can use to help you more consistently expect success.

Change the Experience

If you don't believe in your ability to do something, having a contradictory experience of success can sometimes be jarring enough to dismantle your negative beliefs. Your self-talk influences the way you interpret your experiences. You can have what looks to an objective observer like a success, but through the lens of your perceptions and your critical self-talk, you distort or neutralize it so that it has no impact except to reinforce your negative beliefs. For example, as a tennis player, you've been sporting a 20-match losing streak in which you have consistently played far below your potential. Finally, you get your game back and play well, only to lose a hard-fought match in a tie-breaker. Your coach is thrilled with how well you played. You're devastated! Despite the fact that you played well, you misinterpret the loss as just *another* bad performance because you didn't win. According to your self-talk, nothing's changed. You're still in a slump.

Sometimes, however, an experience can be so powerful that even your trusted way of distorting it to fit your negative beliefs doesn't work. That one experience of success completely obliterates the negative beliefs you held, so that your self-talk has no choice but to change to the positive.

For example, Sergei was a high school miler who had stopped believing in himself and his ability to ever break the five-minute barrier. As a senior, he had run his first five races in the mile between 5:01 and 5:05, and no matter what he tried, he just couldn't seem to go any faster. His junior year had been no different, as his times hovered around 5:02 for both the indoor and outdoor track seasons. His coach had tried everything possible to convince his runner to believe in himself, recognizing that Sergei's lack of belief was the key element in his remaining stuck.

Frustrated by Sergei's lack of response, his coach did something very unusual. In Sergei's sixth race of the year, a dual meet, he ran a 5:02, winning the race by a good 25 yards. As Sergei was crossing the finish line, and *before* he could get his official time, his coach ran out onto the field jumping up and down, celebrating, and screaming "Sergei baby! 4:59!! 4:59!! You finally did it! You finally broke the barrier!" Actually, Sergei's coach had a little pre-race chat with the opposing team's coach, and both had agreed that if Sergei won easily, they would falsify his time. When Sergei left the meet that day, he thought that he *had* broken the barrier. The "evidence" of his "4:59" forced him to abandon his old belief of "I'm just a five-minute miler." He could no longer muster up any negative self-talk about how he'd never be able to do it.

Beliefs directly motivate behavior. When you believe something, you're compelled to take action. The next day, Sergei arrived 45 minutes early for practice and stayed an extra hour. Fueled by his new belief, Sergei continued to show up early and leave late. Four days later in the next dual meet,

Sergei ran an actual 4:58 in the mile. Three days later he ran a 4:59, and for the remainder of his senior year, he consistently broke his old barrier. It was Sergei's new belief, rather than a sudden increase in speed or strength, that caused his breakthrough.

Sergei's situation was indeed unusual and completely set up by his coach. What can *you* do to deliberately change experience yourself? Tough question. Most of the time you'll find this quite difficult. If you're stuck in a

The **Northwestern University football program** was steeped in tradition. Just as Notre Dame and the University of Michigan have long and storied football histories, so Northwestern had a lengthy football tradition—losing. Before 1995 "Loser U," as it was

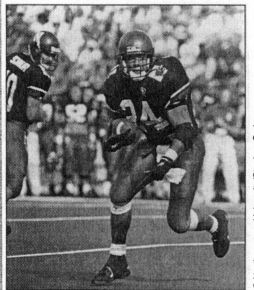
© Northwestern University/Stephen Serio

commonly called, had not had a winning season in 24 years. From their last winning season in 1971 to the start of the 1995 season, the Wildcats averaged two wins a year for 23 years. From 1976 to 1981 Northwestern's record was 3-62-1. During this time the Wildcats made headlines for a 34-game slump over three years that put them in the record books for the longest skid in Division I-A history.

As one could expect, this repetitive long-term failure built strong negative expectations within the athletes and the team. Losing became commonplace and inevitable, creating an almost unstoppable downward momentum that drained confidence and choked off any hope of winning. The only belief that Northwestern's football players had was the inevitability of their failure.

Then in 1992 Northwestern hired a new coach, Gary Barnett. An assistant at Colorado during their program's rebuilding (Colorado was 1-10 in 1984 and national champion by 1990), Barnett was a good coach who had the ability to get his athletes to believe in him and in themselves.

During Barnett's first three years at Northwestern, he seemed no different than all the coaches before him who had promised to finally turn things around but ended up mired in the ongoing futility that was Wildcat football. In 1992 Northwestern went 3-8 and then followed that start with 2-9 and 3-7-1 the next two seasons. However, what outsiders couldn't see was that Barnett was following a plan for success that he had brought with him when he first came to Northwestern. Foremost in this plan was to change the Wildcats' beliefs about themselves and their program.

Barnett started each preseason with a retreat to help his players get away from the self-fulfilling negativity that surrounded them, to build team spirit, and to fill his players' heads with his can-do philosophy. He waged a battle on their self-doubts and taught them to expect success no matter what. This included doing incredibly corny things like singing the old song "High Hopes" as loud as they could. His players slowly began to respond to his positive beliefs and his determination to succeed.

The Wildcats started the 1995 season away at Notre Dame and stunned the college football world with a 17-15 upset victory. Interestingly enough, Barnett didn't view the win as an upset. Long before the season started, he had told his players not to carry him off the field *after* they beat Notre Dame at their place for the first time in 34 years.[1] The Wildcats then went on to beat Michigan and Penn State, two national football powerhouses. Despite each unbelievable win, the Wildcats were seen as a fluke and were still continually picked as the underdog, even against unranked teams. Riding their team play and expectations of success, they continued to mow down the opposition both on the field and in the media. They finished the season 10-1, won the Big Ten championship, and played in the Rose Bowl for the national championship. Despite a 41-32 Rose Bowl loss to USC, the Wildcats finished the 1995 season as big winners.

In 1996 Barnett and Northwestern continued their unexpected winning ways. They went 10-1 over the regular season, were co-champions of the Big Ten, and again qualified for a bowl game, the Citrus Bowl. While they came up short in their postseason efforts, it's clear that Northwestern football has turned belief into reality. Coach Barnett's formula for success was not based on having an overabundance of talent, but on creating a close team who had an unshakable belief in themselves, their coach, and their program.[2]

slump, you can't simply snap out of it by saying to yourself, "No problem! Today I'll just go play out of my mind." If that's all it took to bust out of a slump, like the dinosaurs, these performance problems would have become extinct long ago.

What you can do to shake up those self-limiting beliefs is to continually put yourself in situations that challenge these personal myths. Practice doing the impossible daily. If the basis of your negative beliefs really isn't true, then much of what you tell yourself is impossible, isn't. By attempting the "impossible" over and over, you'll start to take away some of the power of these self-limiting beliefs.

> **B**y attempting the "impossible" over and over, you'll start to take away some of the power of these self-limiting beliefs.

For example, if you're *sure* that you can't train at a certain intensity or run a particular distance, challenge these beliefs and start training harder and running farther. Make yourself get comfortable being uncomfortable. If you believe that you can't execute a certain move on bars or floor, can't land a double axel, or can't rip a reverse dive, continue to take action in the face of these beliefs. That is, attempt the moves, jump, or dive over and over again, forcing yourself to keep practicing them. You can also challenge limiting beliefs outside of sports while tackling your performance difficulties. Sometimes you can knock a brick out of your negative belief structure by first challenging "easier" negative beliefs (like speaking in front of a crowd) or beliefs that aren't as emotionally charged as those involving your performance difficulties, before going after the harder ones.

While changing experience to weaken limiting beliefs is not as easy to do *by yourself* as the other strategies I'm about to show you, it may be the fastest if you can get the right experience. As a coach, you can have a significant impact on your athletes' beliefs by facilitating positive experiences.

In an old Walt Disney cartoon classic about Dumbo, the flying elephant, Dumbo does not believe that he can fly until a crow gives him a magic feather. With the magic feather in his trunk, Dumbo is convinced that he can fly and, as a result of his belief, he does so. This is nothing new to successful coaches. They have been handing out these magic feathers to their athletes since the dawn of sport.

For example, coaches at every level regularly say and do things to alter athletes' experiences and get them to believe in themselves. A swim coach, at a loss to explain his women's team's poor performance in the morning of a two-day meet, told them *with the certainty of an expert* that the main reason they swam badly was iron deficiency. His remedy? Over the lunch break, he took them to a local drug store to buy vitamins. After they took the vitamins, they swam some of their best performances.

Similarly, a basketball coach told a talented fifth grader that the secret to improving her free throws was to be sure to always have the air valve on the ball to her right whenever she stepped to the line. When this player went on to set a high school record for most points scored in her state, she continued to *believe* that "valve placement" was critical to her success at the foul line, even though intellectually she knew it really didn't matter.

As another example, a high school wrestling coach regularly had his athletes "practice" the experience of winning. At his whistle, practice would stop, Olympic theme music would be turned on, and his entire team would gather over by the awards platform. One wrestler would then climb up to the top step and the entire team and coaching staff would cheer this athlete as if he had just won a major tournament. When NCAA and two-time world champion wrestler Lee Kemp was just beginning in the sport, he built an awards platform in his room and practiced these feelings of being number one.

Change Self-Talk

The next major building block in the belief structure is self-talk. You can attack negative beliefs by directly going after the underlying self-talk. Self-talk maintains negative beliefs by coloring your experiences in a certain way. If you can change the self-talk attached to your experiences, you'll weaken the hold that those negative beliefs have over you. Once this happens, you'll then be positioned to replace performance-disrupting beliefs with more positive ones.

> **B**y changing the self-talk attached to your experiences, you'll weaken the hold that negative beliefs have over you.

Changing self-talk begins with awareness. You must recognize the negative chatter that reinforces these negative beliefs. ("Here we go again. I always choke under pressure. I'll never get this. I didn't play like that last year. What's wrong with me? She's so much better than I am. I don't have a chance.") Look back to your answers to the "What Mental Strategies Are You Using?" exercise in Step 2 on pages 27-28, where you identified your slump-fueling self-talk. Once you've developed this awareness, you want to interrupt the negative flow and replace it with more positive inner coaching. Do not expect yourself to believe this new self-talk in the beginning. Your doubting of this new voice is actually the first step in the process of changing a negative belief into a positive one. Be persistent with the following exercises, and soon the walls of those negative beliefs will start to crumble.

Change the Time Frame. One common characteristic of slumping athletes' self-talk is their use of words that convey a message of *permanence* about their performance difficulties: "This is the way things have *been*, and this is how they'll *always* be." "Permanent" language in your self-talk kills your confidence and fuels a sense of hopelessness.

For example, a pitcher with major league potential is struggling with control problems. He throws two balls in the dirt and starts thinking, "*Whenever* I get in these pressure situations, this *always* seems to happen to me. I can throw great in the bullpen, but I just *can't* throw well when it counts!" The language in his self-talk carries with it an air of permanence, of unchangeability. It basically says "your problems are here to stay."

When you talk to yourself using the language of permanence, you feed the negative beliefs that keep you stuck. The team that thinks "we can *never* win the big game" or "we *always* choke under pressure" demonstrates a similar self-defeating quality of permanence in their language. The golfer who thinks to himself, "I *can't* make three-foot putts" or "I have no short game" after double-bogeying a big hole is mentally leaving himself no way out. He is unknowingly creating an illusion of permanence.

It is interesting that great athletes like Michael Jordan, Joe Montana, Bonnie Blair, and Jackie Joyner-Kersee use a similar kind of permanence

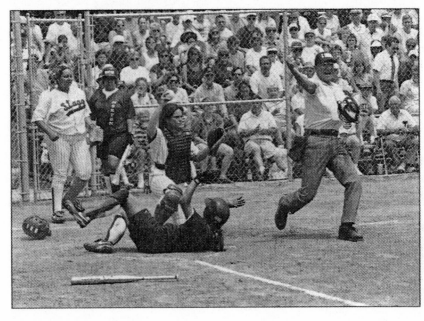

© Human Kinetics

in the language of their self-talk. However, in their cases, this permanence is used to reinforce a positive belief (for example, "I want the ball at crunch time because I *always* know what to do," "*Whenever* my back's to the wall, I excel," and "I *can* do it."). This is exactly what happens to you when you're "on" or "in the zone." You step to the line to serve with your team down by five points in the deciding game of the tournament, and you think, "All right! I love these situations. I *always* play well under pressure. I have hit some of my best serves when the game is on the line. I *never* mess up when it counts."

To shake the foundation on which those slump-fueling negative beliefs rest, you must monitor and then *change* your use of permanent language. When you lose your balance, stumble, and fall, you must describe this to yourself in a temporary way. For example, "Boy, was I off *today!*" "What a terrible match that was; *tomorrow* will be better," and "I can't do that *yet*" all convey a *time-limited, changeable* quality. Similarly, telling yourself, "I was tired," "I didn't feel well," or "I was just off; it was one of those days" reflects a temporariness that does not contribute to the development of negative beliefs.

You should monitor your use of negativity and permanent language mainly during a break in practice or after competition. Don't distract yourself *while* you are performing with this analytical focus. Being too much in your head at competition time is part of the problem contributing to the slump, so we don't want you thinking *more* when you compete. The thought-stopping technique discussed later in this step is more appropriate for handling negative self-talk *during* competition.

Start to look at your failures and mistakes *not* as a continuation of a never-ending process, but as a *temporary* and *time-limited deviation* from your normal good performance. When you carry statistics in your head and drag the past into the present (for example, "I haven't had a great race in over eight months," "That's the sixth easy putt I've missed this round," and "How many times do I choke when it counts?"), you create an illusion of permanence that keeps you slumping.

Once in the dugout before a game, baseball great Willie Mays told everyone, "This is going to be a great day. I'm going 4 for 4 today. No doubt about it!" After Mays struck out his first time up, he came back to the dugout with a smile on his face and said, "This is a great day today. . .I'm going 3 for 4!" In his second at-bat, Mays flied out to the left fielder. Back in the dugout he told his teammates, "I'm going 2 for 4 today!" Later in the game when he grounded out to the shortstop for his third at-bat, he said, "I'm going 1 for 4 today. . .and that's a fact." When he was robbed of a base hit by the right fielder in his last at-bat of the day, Mays told his teammates, " Tomorrow is going to be a great day. I'm going 4 for 4!"

Mays's attitude reflected the temporary quality necessary for busting slumps and staying out of their nasty clutches. If you're going to use permanent language in your self-talk, confine it to explaining your successes ("I always play well here," or "I'm the best athlete in this competition.").

> ***L**ook at your failures not as a continuation of a never-ending process, but as a temporary deviation from your normal good performance.*

If you're slumping, *stop* explaining away your victories in *temporary* terms ("It was a fluke. I was lucky. I never hit that well."). This further feeds your negative beliefs. To get in the habit of changing the time frame of your self-talk, using temporary language to explain your failures and permanent language to explain your successes, complete the following exercises and then carry them with you through practice and competition.

Reframe Negative Beliefs. Another good way to practice turning negative beliefs into positive ones is through reframing or the "lemonade strategy." I briefly introduced the technique of reframing in Step 4 as a way of mastering fears. This strategy can also help you weaken the grip of negative beliefs by deliberately altering the underlying self-talk. The lemonade strategy is based on the axiom, "When life deals you lemons, make lemonade."

As an athlete, you always have two options when adversity is thrown your way. First, you can bemoan your fate and curse the performance gods for their cruelty. This is what happens when you focus on the adversity and

MAKING YOUR SETBACKS TEMPORARY

The left column contains examples of negative self-talk following a failure or setback. This self-talk reflects a permanent time frame and feeds negative beliefs. By altering the wording, make each sentence reflect a more temporary explanation of the failure or mistake. Sample answers appear at the end of the exercise.

■ Permanent

■ Temporary

Example:

Why can't I ever swim fast when it counts?

I had a really bad race this morning.

1. We always blow the big lead.

2. Whenever I try my best,
   I come up short.
3. The coach never plays me.
4. I just can't do it.
5. They're impossible to beat.
6. I'm a total head case.
7. Our captain is unfair.
8. I can't play in the wind.
9. The referees are blind
   and unfair.
10. Why bother; coach never
    listens to me anyway.

The following sample answers represent only one of many ways that you could rephrase each statement in "temporary" terms.

1. We had a chance to win today and let up. We gave them one too many chances.
2. I gave it everything I had, but it wasn't enough today.
3. The coach needed the hot hitters in the lineup today.
4. I haven't been able to do it yet.
5. They have a good team, but we really improved in practices this week.
6. I let my nerves get the better of me this time.
7. The captain made an unfair call in that situation.
8. The wind distracted me today.
9. The refs made a bad call on that play.
10. I'm not sure coach heard what I said; perhaps I need to say it differently next time.

use it as an excuse for your failure (for example, "It was just too windy today," "No wonder I did so bad; I had to compete last in the rotation. What a ripoff!" and "The refs were like the three blind mice today!"). Second, you can "make lemonade" out of those uncontrollable "lemons" that were thrown at you. That is, you can use adversity to boost your confidence and intensity. This option is what we recommended in our discussion of handling performance uncontrollables in Step 2—use them as your competitive edge.

MAKING YOUR SUCCESSES PERMANENT

In the following examples of self-talk used to explain away a slumping athlete's successes, change the language from temporary to permanent. Sample answers appear at the end of the exercise.

■ Temporary

■ Permanent

Example:

We were so lucky to win.

We play really well together.

1. No wonder I won;
   I had no competition.

2. Yeah, but he sprained
   his ankle in the tie-breaker,
   which is why I made it to
   the next round.

3. My opponent got kind
   of tired at the end.

4. No one really saw me coming;
   otherwise, I doubt that I
   would've been able to sneak
   in and score.

5. (jokingly) We paid the
   refs off; that's why we won.

6. They just weren't used to
   playing in front of such a
   large crowd and we were.

7. Someone was watching out
   for me today. Talk about
   freak occurrences!

8. Their best player couldn't
   play today.

9. Our defense got lucky.

10. The judges were a lot harder
    on the earlier competitors
    than they were on me.

The following sample answers represent only one of many ways that you could explain the success in permanent terms.

1. I won because I trained hard and was ready. I deserved this victory.
2. Even though he sprained his ankle, I was giving him the toughest match he'd ever had. I belong in this round.
3. I'm in fantastic condition.
4. My game plan was perfect and it wouldn't have mattered what my competition knew or didn't know I was planning.
5. We're a better, more disciplined, closer team. . .and we wanted it more.
6. We know how to stay cool under big-game pressure.
7. I made the breaks I got today. I create my own luck.
8. We can beat anyone they run out there.
9. We have a tough team and our defense is awesome!
10. The judges know a class act when they see it.

For example, questionable calls from the referees are an uncontrollable. Being angry with the officials or arguing with them will rarely improve your play. Instead, it will mentally (and frequently physically) take you out of the game. The Chicago Bulls' eccentric star rebounder Dennis Rodman was so upset with a call during a game in March 1996 that he lost his cool and head-butted a referee. Rodman was immediately suspended for six games and fined $20,000.

Use adversity to boost your confidence and intensity.

Rather than dwelling on the bad call and getting bitter, learn to make lemonade. This might entail thinking to yourself, "The refs are an uncontrollable, and if I focus on them, I'm going to lose it. I'll use every bad call as a signal to focus even more intensely. I also know that the bad calls are going to bother my opponents more than me." Reframing questionable calls in this way will keep your confidence high and help you stay mentally in the game.

In the heat of competition, opponents will sometimes resort to behaviors that exceed the rules of fair play. They will talk trash, play overly aggressively, or blatantly cheat. Their behaviors may push your buttons and get you to react without thinking. If you learn to control your self-talk in these situations and reframe your opponent's behavior (for example, "She's not feeling good enough about her own skills to beat me fairly, so she has to resort to cheating."), you'll feel more confident about the situation and more in control.

Stop Negative Thoughts.   Turning negative self-talk into a more positive dialogue will ultimately weaken the negative beliefs that keep you stuck. Thought-stopping is a skill you can practice in training and before competition. The five-stage process listed on page 122 will help you first recognize that you're entertaining negativity, and then interrupt it and turn it around in a positive way.

MAKING LEMONADE

Use the lemonade strategy to reframe the following examples of negative self-talk. Sometimes you may have to really stretch your thinking to come up with anything positive. If you're currently stuck in a slump, you're probably well-practiced in being negative. Trying to find the positive reframe may be difficult at first. Don't worry if you don't believe the reframe immediately. Just get in the habit of making lemonade. Be creative here to find the opportunity hidden in the problem. Sample answers appear at the end of the exercise.

Original	Reframed
Examples:	
Their crowd is in your face the whole game. They really give that team an unfair advantage.	We can gain the upper hand by taking their crowd right out of the game. All we have to do is focus on our plan and use the heckling as a reminder to stay calm and do our job.
I hate playing in the wind.	The wind is going to upset my opponent more than me. I can use it to get an edge.

1. What a terrible mistake to make! And so early in the contest. It's gonna be one of those days.

2. They are so much taller than we are.

3. This crowd is really huge!

4. They have two all-conference athletes on their squad. We're in big trouble.

5. It's so cold I can barely feel my hands and feet. How can the coach possibly expect us to play in this weather?

6. She's beaten me six races in a row. Why should today be any different?

7. I feel so tired and broken down. I know I'm not going to play well.

8. This is going to be some of the worst officiating you'll ever see in your life.

9. Their school's bigger. They have more scholarships than we do. They have better training facilities. We haven't a prayer.

10. Just my luck. We're all set to play and now we have this delay! Why does this always happen to me?

The following sample answers represent one of many possible ways to reframe the negative self-talk.

1. No problem. Now that I've got that mistake out of the way I can really relax and look forward to playing well the rest of the game.

2. We're faster and smarter and will catch them off guard.

3. This is a great opportunity to practice staying focused.

4. What a great opportunity to show what we can do against such good athletes. They probably won't take us seriously, which will really work to our benefit.

5. This cold is great. Look at what it's doing to everyone else's concentration. I can just relax now and use the cold to focus me even more.

6. Today is a new race. She looks over-confident. She's definitely got more to lose than I do here.

7. Everyone else on that field is as tired as I am, so now it's a question of who is the toughest mentally. That's me, without a doubt.

8. Since we know the calls are going to be outrageous, we can ignore them and focus on our game.

9. Because we have had to work harder with less, we're much tougher than they are. Are they ever in for a surprise!

10. This is great! Everybody hates delays and I can use this time to relax and focus. Let everyone else stress out over it.

1. Recognize the negativity as quickly as possible.
2. Say "stop" loudly to yourself.
3. Take a slow, deep breath, imagining that, as you exhale, you can breathe the negativity far away from you.
4. Reframe the negative thought into a positive one or change the time frame of the thought from permanent to temporary.
5. Refocus your concentration on the task at hand.

As an example, pretend you have just missed an uncontested lay-up in the waning seconds of a basketball game that would have given your team the victory (or use a similar example from your sport). Because of your miss, the game is now going into overtime. Before the overtime period, your self-talk is excessively critical, "I can't believe you missed that shot. You always let the team down. What a choke! Why can't you come through for once!" If you stay with this kind of internal punishment, you'll be too nervous, distracted, and unsure of yourself to play well. In the few seconds that remain before the game resumes, your use of the thought-stopping technique might resemble the following example.

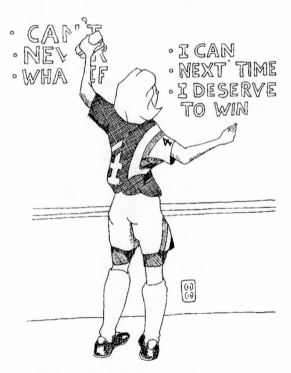

Change your self-talk.

Recognizing that you're emotionally pounding on yourself (stage 1), you think, "Whoa! Stop!!" (stage 2). You then take a slow, deep breath, imagining you can breathe away all that mental garbage (stage 3). Next, you deliberately turn the negative chatter to positive by thinking, "You've played a great game so far. Your defense has been solid and you're already on the board for 15 points. Forget it. . .let it go. . .get back in the game." (stage 4). Finally, as you walk out onto the court, you put your focus of concentration on executing the planned play after the tip-off (stage 5).

You can use a number of streamlined variations of thought-stopping in practice or in competition. The effectiveness of these techniques lies in your ability to recognize the negativity quickly and interrupt it before it can pull disruptive emotions from you. Such an ability will only come from putting in enough time practicing the techniques that seem to fit for you. Sufficient practice makes it easier to be on top of the negativity and effectively change it.

The thought-stopping techniques can be used before practice or games and even during the contests. You may find, however, that consciously fighting with your negativity is a distraction. For example, if negative self-talk pops up just as you bring the club face back to putt, as you toss the ball in the air for your serve, or as the signals are being called on the line, the very last thing you want to do is begin an internal fight. In these situations

THOUGHT-STOPPING VARIATIONS

The following strategies are variations of the thought-stopping technique just presented. All entail streamlined versions of the five-stage process, using either a physical action or some form of imagery:

- The Rubber Band—Put an elastic band on your wrist, and every time you become aware of a negative thought, snap the band against your wrist. The sudden quick pain will "snap you out" of the negativity and remind you to get your focus back in the practice or game. Note: If you begin to notice lacerations resulting from the repeated use of this technique, discontinue immediately.

- Exhale—Imagine that you have a pipe-like connection between your brain and lungs. Just by exhaling, you can eliminate any negative self-talk that arises, as if your exhalation were an exhaust pipe. You can inhale relaxation and calming thoughts and exhale negativity.

- Erase It—Imagine that you can take the negative self-talk and write it on a piece of paper or a chalkboard. Take an eraser and rub out

→

the negative writing until it disappears completely from your mind's eye. Bruce Lee used to imagine writing his negative self-talk on a piece of paper, crumbling the paper up, and then setting fire to it.

- Change the Channel—Imagine that you can create an image of the negative self-talk as if it were on a TV screen. Change the channel or otherwise blur the screen so that the picture with the writing becomes unreadable.

- Turn the Volume Down—Hear the negative self-talk as if it were on a radio or CD player and then turn the volume down until you can no longer make out the words. As you turn the volume down on the negative chatter, you can even replace it by gradually increasing the volume on music of your choice until this music ultimately drowns out the negativity.

- Be an Opera Singer—Imagine that you are a famous opera singer. Sing the negative self-talk in an operatic voice (to yourself, please). You may find that it is extremely difficult to take your negativity seriously when you hear it presented in this manner.

thought-stopping is too cumbersome and distracting a technique to use. Instead, learn to refocus your concentration and play through the negativity.

Develop Positive Affirmations. You don't believe in yourself. You feel that you don't belong on the team. You're not at all sure that you'll ever break out of your performance doldrums. Your negative self-talk brings you down and fuels your slump. One way to interrupt this negativity and break down the walls of self-limiting beliefs is by using *affirmations*. An affirmation is a positive self-statement that you focus on and repeat to yourself many times a day. The power behind this technique is found in the adage, "You become what you think about most of the time." Few athletes can really believe an affirmation the first time they use it. With repeated practice, however, the positive self-statement starts to take hold.

For example, as a freshman, Amy was a talented high school hockey player who entertained a nagging belief that she somehow didn't fit in. She didn't think she was very good and felt that she had no impact on the squad. She was excessively self-critical and continually interpreted situations so that she would feel bad. Her negativity and lack of confidence spilled over into her schoolwork and social life.

To help Amy begin to dislodge her self-limiting beliefs, we used affirmations. She found the first one that we developed for her, "I am a positive, confident force," rather amusing, given that it was the *exact oppo-*

site of how she really felt. When developing an affirmation, write down how you'd like to feel and what you'd like to believe *as if it were true right now*. Like Amy's, your affirmations should stretch the limits of your present beliefs.

Affirmations should stretch the limits of your beliefs.

Amy was then given the homework assignment to write this affirmation on a number of index cards and tape them in visible places all around her house. For example, Amy taped a card to the ceiling over her bed, so her affirmation was the last thing she saw before sleep and the first thing she saw when she opened her eyes in the morning. She put them on her walls, mirror, and refrigerator. I instructed her to take them to school; put them in her notebooks, locker, and desk; and look at them throughout the day. She wrote the affirmation on her hockey stick, gloves, pads, and even on the back of her hand. A few weeks later, she reported that she was feeling a little better about herself and that being a "positive, confident force" didn't seem so silly to her anymore. She related several instances on the ice and in the classroom when she actually felt that she was that "force."

Use the following examples to practice turning your negative feelings into positive affirmations:

Negative Feeling	Positive Affirmation
I choke under pressure.	I always come through in the clutch.
I have zero confidence in myself.	I'm a confident, self-assured winner.
When things go badly, I fall apart.	When the going gets rough, I hang tough.
I feel totally out of control.	I am always in control, the master of my destiny.
I can't perform when I'm tired.	I have unlimited endurance.

Like most techniques discussed in this book, those that will help you change negative self-talk require consistent and committed practice. Making lemonade, changing the time frame, thought-stopping, or using affirmations will only work for you if you work at them.

Change Your Actions

Beliefs impel people to take action. The action is visible in a person's behaviors on a gross-motor level in movement and on a micro-motor level in facial expression, breathing, and posture. These behaviors then touch off certain emotions that are an outward reflection of the person's inner beliefs. If you believe something to be true, you're likely to follow that belief with observable action and behaviors that support it.

> **I**f you believe something, you're likely to follow that belief
> with observable actions that support it.

For example, you're in a slump and have stopped believing in yourself. Things have gotten so bad that you're even beginning to question whether you'll ever get unstuck. Your outward behaviors reflect this belief. When you step up to the plate, you act as if you have no confidence. You drag your feet slightly. Your head and shoulders sag a little. Your facial expression is a dead giveaway of your nervousness and self-doubts. Everything about your physical actions and posture outwardly mirror the self-limiting beliefs that you hold inwardly.

Furthermore, by acting as if you have no faith in yourself, you end up feeling even less confident. Outwardly acting like you don't think you can reinforces those emotions inside and makes it even more likely that you won't. Your physical actions, posture, and facial expression all have a significant impact in *generating* your emotions. Your emotions, in turn, reinforce your beliefs. Another way to go about changing self-limiting beliefs is to change your actions or behaviors.

It's a commonly held notion that *if* you feel confident, you'll *then* act this way—the inner emotions generate the outer behaviors. Dr. James Laird from Clark University in Worcester, Massachusetts did a classic study that demonstrated just the opposite—that it's your outer behaviors, particularly facial expressions, that generate your inner feelings. Dr. Laird took his subjects in a room and gave them instructions about how to very subtly change their facial expressions (for example, raise your left eyebrow slightly, lower the right side of your mouth, etc.). When he was finished with these directions, the subjects unknowingly had made their faces look scared, mad, glad, or depressed. After maintaining this facial position for a certain amount of time, the subjects were then asked to respond to a questionnaire designed to determine their present emotional state. He discovered that the subject's emotions directly reflected their facial expressions and that the specific facial expression generated the inner feelings that the subject reported.

The mental strategy of acting as if naturally reflects the outcome of Dr. Laird's study. Acting as if is based on the principle that your emotions or how you feel on the inside are always determined by how you act on the outside. Therefore, you can learn to change your emotional state just by altering your behaviors, posture, and facial expression. Changing these minibehaviors will shift the beliefs that are fed by the emotions. Acting as if is very simply the idea that if you *act* the way that you want to become, you'll become the way you act.

Acting as if has absolutely nothing to do with talking a good game. If you believe you're a head case, acting as if has nothing to do with telling anyone within earshot that you're the best athlete ever in your sport. Instead, acting as if is a deliberate and nonverbal attempt to alter your body physiology (breathing, posture, facial expression, and movement), so that you pretend to be the way that you want to be. It's been said that *you can master anything that you can pretend.*

Acting as if can be considered a winner's fall-back position. That is, a mentally tough athlete who is feeling intimidated will act as if she's confident. She will hold her head up, move calmly, and smile. If she's exhausted, this athlete will act as if she has a lot of energy by jumping around or moving strongly and powerfully. It is interesting how lying around when you're really tired makes you feel even more exhausted. Acting as if is simply known as the "fake-it-till-you-make-it" strategy.

But when you're in the performance dumpster, how do you act otherwise? How can you really apply this strategy in a way that will be useful to you? Start by making a deliberate attempt to be more aware of how you carry yourself in practice and at competition. When things go poorly for you, how does your posture tend to change? What about your facial expression? You must take this awareness and deliberately act the opposite of how you are feeling. When you're feeling blue, you must consciously start to fake it, regardless of how silly you feel. Put a smile on your face. Slow and deepen your breathing. Pick your head and shoulders up. Walk with a spring in your step and start acting like a winner. If you can get in the habit of acting as if, you'll begin to nullify the negative emotions and weaken the impact of those self-limiting beliefs.

Ignore the Experts

In 1954, runner Roger Bannister did the impossible, breaking the four-minute barrier in the mile with a 3:59. At the time of Bannister's feat, the "experts" had all stated that it was physically impossible for the human body to withstand the strain of running that fast. Bannister was a medical student at the time and there were even published medical reports that supported this limiting belief. Beliefs control behavior. They will either propel you toward a goal or hold you back, depending on what you believe. Beliefs are frequently established by the "experts" in the field.

After Bannister broke the barrier, a number of runners followed suit. A year later, all eight runners in one race recorded sub–four-minute times.

And just a few years later Jim Ryan, a high schooler, broke the "impossible" barrier as well. So much for experts! If you're presently in a slump, are there any "experts" who may be directly or indirectly feeding your performance difficulties? Surrounding yourself with supportive friends, coaches, and family is absolutely critical to help you break free. However, you don't want any experts on your team who tend to rain on your parade. These individuals may mean well, but their "for-your-own-good" brand of negativity will keep you stuck and poison your motivation. For example, parents may not want to see their kid suffer anymore or fail again, so they encourage him to stop trying. Or a friend who isn't comfortable taking risks herself encourages you to play it safe. The only experts you want on your team are those who believe in you *no matter what*.

Choose carefully whose beliefs you're going to adopt. Be sure that they help you get back on track. If you have a vote of confidence from a trusted coach who hasn't stopped believing in you while you've been struggling, it will be much easier for you to turn your own self-doubts around.

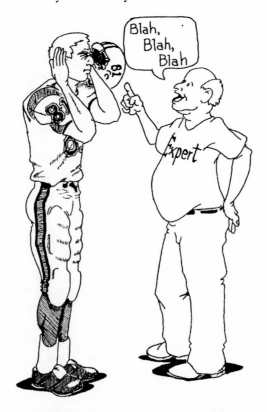

Don't listen to the experts.

Associate to Past Successes

Over the course of a career, sooner or later every athlete runs into a road-block or two. You may get temporarily knocked off track, slowed down, or completely stuck by these. For example, getting cut from a team, suffering a disappointing loss, sustaining a serious injury, reaching a plateau, or being blocked by fears can all generate beliefs that can keep you stuck. As you think about your career, can you remember a time when you felt stuck and seriously questioned yourself? Can you think back to how you successfully overcame those self-limiting beliefs? Can you remember a time when you felt ready to pack it all in, yet you somehow mustered enough strength and reserve to overcome that obstacle and change your belief?

*P*ast successes are resources for the slumping athlete.

These past successes are hidden resources for the slumping athlete. Within these old experiences are the resources that you may need *today* to overcome that slump. By remembering in detail a time when you were able to extricate yourself from an "impossible" situation, you can get back in touch with your personal strengths and abilities.

Learn From Other Athletes

If you're stuck, then you've probably lost your perspective. You may be so caught up with the problem that the idea of a *solution* may be the farthest thing from your mind. Consequently, you may not be able to see a way out. Seeing no way out will leave you feeling isolated. You may think "why me?" and feel like you're the only one who has ever struggled. To counter-act your isolation and begin to turn around those negative beliefs, track down and interview other athletes who have successfully overcome similar slumps.

Ask your coach, teammates, or local sportswriters if they know anyone, amateur or professional, who has had to overcome the adversity that is currently haunting you. If you can't come up with any "live" examples, go to your local library and find some books written about successful athletes or individuals outside of sports who at one time or another during their careers endured painful slumps. Some examples include Sadahara Oh, author of *A Zen Way of Baseball*; Tim Daggett, author of *Dare to Dream*; and Norman Cousins, author of *Anatomy of an Illness*.

Talking to or reading about other athletes who have struggled and over-come their slumps will give you a better perspective (slumps happen to every kind of athlete), a renewed sense of hope (slumps actually can have a happy ending), and some very practical strategies to help get yourself unstuck. Reading about or talking to these "pioneers" who have successfully gone before you may make it a little easier for you to believe in yourself again. As you begin to believe in yourself, your performance expectations will change. You may even be surprised to find yourself once again expecting success the way the "old, preslump you" did long ago.

Conclusion

Your athletic performance is truly self-fulfilling. You will get what you *expect*. The techniques in this step have been designed to teach you how to break down negative, self-limiting beliefs and replace them with more positive ones. By deliberately and consistently changing your experience, self-talk, and behaviors, you will diminish the slump's power over you.

As you begin to believe in yourself once more and expect success, you'll notice that these expectations are accompanied by a positive change in your inner "movies." When you are in a slump and expecting failure, your inner images preview this failure. Before your competition, you envision yourself making mistakes and your performance falling. With a change in your beliefs, you now begin to see what you *want to happen* instead of what you're *afraid will happen*. Suddenly you can see yourself making the catch, getting a clutch hit, posting a best time, or making the team. In the next step of the slump-busting model, we will teach you how to further develop and enhance these positive images.

STEP
6
DEVELOPING
POSITIVE IMAGES

"Winners see what they want to have happen while losers see what they are afraid will happen."

When successful athletes "think" about an upcoming game, their thinking is often accompanied by internal pictures, an internal "feel" of the muscle movements, and internal sounds. These inner images, feelings, and sounds are consistent with the results that they seek. They mentally experience themselves running well, executing the plays as planned, feeling confident, and effectively handling the pressure. When this thinking is done deliberately, it's called *mental rehearsal* or *visualization*. Some athletes purposely set aside practice time to mentally preview exactly how they would like to perform. For others, this process happens automatically and unconsciously. While these athletes may tell you that they do not knowingly practice mental rehearsal, their positive thinking about the upcoming event generates performance-enhancing internal imagery.

Slumping athletes, on the other hand, do not have positive images of the performance the night before and day of the big game. While they try to think positively and see what they want to happen, their thoughts and internal imagery consistently gravitate to the negative. They see themselves fumbling the ball in the end zone, getting out-touched to lose the race, striking out with the bases loaded, or missing the game-saving free throws. Why? Are slumping athletes masochists who enjoy watching their own version of the agony of defeat? Absolutely not! They desperately want to

131

stop singing the performance blues, but they just can't get that tune out of their heads.

No matter how hard slumping athletes try to picture themselves gracefully walking on water, they keep coming up with images of swallowing a tubful and sinking to the bottom. Their thinking and internal imagery are almost reflexively pulled in a negative direction. They either see what they want the *least* or experience the screen going blank at crucial moments. For some slumping athletes, the issue isn't negative images; it's simply no images at all! In the 1984 Olympics, American Mary Decker Slaney was tripped in the later stages of the 10,000-meter run by South African Zola Budd and was unable to finish the race. In a postrace interview, Mary claimed that while she had mentally rehearsed the race many times before the Olympics, she *never* saw herself finishing in any of her mental practices!

Y*ou can't bust that slump if your preperformance viewing continually depicts you making mistakes.*

If you're currently struggling as an athlete, your next step in the slump-busting model after attacking your fears and learning to defeat negative beliefs is to change your choice of inner movies. You can't bust that slump if your preperformance viewing continually depicts you making mistakes. Like athletes at the top of their game, you must learn to see yourself succeed. Developing positive images, like many of the steps in this model, is interconnected with other steps and has a profound impact on your entire mental game. As you learn to harness the power of positive images, remember that the slump-busting process combines several or all of the 10 interconnected strategies to eliminate your performance difficulties. How do you know which steps will work best for you? If you have a fear-based performance problem, Step 4 will certainly be relevant. But you'll also find that Step 3's concentration techniques and Step 10's strategies for managing stress will also be useful. Similarly, if your slump has left you feeling negative, incompetent, and expecting failure, Step 5's techniques for expecting success and Step 8's strategies for building confidence will be important to you. Because the effects of one step, for example, developing positive images, will influence several others, it's important that you read the entire book to discover which steps best fit your performance problem and work best for you.

What Movies Are You Watching?

Mike, a struggling touring golf professional, approached his ball in the middle of the fifth fairway, warily checking out the stand of trees some 200 yards away that directly separated him from the green. He had two options. First, he could play his second shot safe and drive the ball straight ahead, just to the right of the woods. This would leave him a direct shot at the green to the left, unimpeded by the trees. Second, he could play the shot more aggressively, the way a pro of his caliber should, going straight over the trees directly for the green. If he played it this way, with a decent shot he'd be on in two with an easy chance at birdie. If he blew it, he'd be in the woods and lucky to get away with a double bogey. I watched him line the shot up, stand over the ball, and then pull the trigger. The ball flew off his club as if it were radar guided, heading straight for the center of the trees. He groaned loudly as it disappeared from view. The ball hit a tree trunk with a solid thump, and Mike disgustedly said, "You know, I *knew* that was going to happen! I *saw* it landing in the center of those stupid trees before I even hit the ball! I don't know why I always seem to prejudge my failures."

Mike's mental mistake of previewing his performance nightmare before it happened is quite common to the slumping athlete. It's not that Mike and athletes like him have a crystal ball and can accurately predict the future; they *create* it. Their negative imagery becomes one of the causes of their performance problems. The quality of your internal imagery directly preprograms your performance. While successful athletes either consciously or unconsciously make pictures in their mind's eye of what they *want to happen* before the action, slumping athletes see what they are *afraid will happen*. Simply put, the inner movies of struggling athletes are terrifying and performance-disrupting.

> *T**he quality of your internal imagery directly preprograms your performance.*

As a gymnast, Amanda had been stuck on a back walkover on the beam for over eight months. Since she could do the trick on both the floor and the low beam (six inches off the ground), she was perfectly capable of executing the skill physically. However, she was too filled with fears to take the skill up to the high beam (four feet off the ground). Whenever she attempted the back walkover on the high beam, she froze and refused to budge until her frustrated coach finally told her to dismount. What stopped her? Was she that afraid of heights? Her problem stemmed from being convinced that if she attempted the skill, she'd miss her hands and hit her head on the beam. While no one in her gym had ever missed her hands and banged her head, Amanda was sure that it *would* happen to her. How could she be so sure? Easy! She could see it happening—clearly and vividly—in her mind's eye whenever she thought about doing the skill. As long as this horror movie continued to play in her mind, she stayed stuck. She was finally able to get over her block after she learned to consistently change the movie and see and feel herself planting her hands firmly on the beam and safely executing the skill.

Slumping athletes' mental imagery is like returning from a video store with what they thought was their own personal "Road to Glory" highlight film, only to discover as the film begins that the clerk had mistakenly given them "Road to Gory" instead. If you play inner horror flicks of yourself crashing and burning just before you perform, you can be sure of several things. First, your anxiety will rise to performance-disrupting heights. Second, your self-confidence will do a serious nosedive. Third, your muscles will tighten sufficiently to make your skill execution unrecognizable. When you step out to perform, filled with tension and self-doubt, you can be sure that your performance will *not* be one for the record books.

So why not just change your selection of these inner movies? Is that such a difficult task? Your natural reaction to these questions may very well be, "Yeah, right. Easier said than done. And it's not like I'm doing this on purpose. I don't exactly enjoy seeing myself humiliated time and time again. It's just that every time I try to picture myself playing well, I always end up screwing things up! It's as if there's someone in my head messing with the projector."

Though you may not *yet* feel it, you *are* in control. The key question here is *how* do you go about getting this control back? In this step you'll learn how to alter your inner movies so that they begin to work *for* instead of *against* you. If we can help you change your inner movie reviews to "four stars," soon your actual performances will merit rave reviews.

The Power of Mental Images

How do your mental images have such a powerful effect on your sports performance? Your internal imagery can serve as a bridge to reality. If you can learn to experience yourself performing optimally in your mind's eye, then soon you'll be able to perform that way in the athletic arena.

The power of mental rehearsal is based on the idea that for short periods of time, your brain can't tell the difference between experiences that are real and those that are *vividly* imagined. You have probably had the experience of waking up from a scary dream, absolutely convinced for a minute or two that the dream was real. Your body had responded to the movie that was playing in your mind with pounding heart and sweaty brow. For a moment you may have anxiously looked around the room, muscles on edge, ready to fight or flee. Similarly, sometimes people get lost in daydreams that are so lifelike that the boundaries of their present reality are temporarily blurred.

When you mentally re-create an experience in vivid detail—seeing, hearing, feeling, and smelling the moment—you experience a similar physiological response. That is, your brain records the experience as if it were actually happening. Your nerves and muscles respond to the imagined performance, and repeated "practice" can actually program your muscles to react in a particular way. Further, the memory of this experience, assuming it is positive, can be used to help you feel calm, confident, and focused the next time you perform. The more you repeatedly imagine something in vivid detail, using all your senses, the easier it is for your body, mind, and emotions to know exactly what to do when you are actually placed in this situation.

Mental rehearsal is a wonderful tool to help you get unstuck or master something that you've never done before. It provides you with a safe vehicle to practice the scary, embarrassing, or difficult without fear of negative consequences. When done right, this inner practice can serve as a valuable weapon to help you break the slump. Depending on the specifics of your performance problem, you can fine-tune the mental rehearsal to go right to the heart of the matter. Like a "smart bomb," your imagery practice can be targeted to obliterate the particular culprit that's been insidiously sabotaging your performance.

Mental rehearsal lets you practice the scary, embarrassing, or difficult without fear of negative consequences.

For example, after more than six months of throwing up before every 200-yard freestyle race she swam in, 12-year-old Beth was finally able to stay calm and relaxed by deliberately using mental rehearsal to change her internal images. Her problem started shortly after she had moved up into a more competitive age group. In her second meet of the season, she became so preoccupied with having to prove herself that she started to experience intense stomach cramps. Because of her discomfort, she was unable to swim well in her best event, the 200 freestyle. This failure left her feeling humiliated.

Her self-imposed pressure to do well and a worry that the stomach problems might happen again caused her to experience the same problems at her next meet. Soon she was staying up nights before meets, panicked by images of having stomach problems and swimming badly. Her worry disrupted her sleep and left her frazzled and nauseated before her races. At the season-ending championships, she got so nervous before her 200 that she vomited just as she was getting up on the blocks for the start. She felt totally humiliated. She was too drained emotionally and physically to compete. She swam the worst race of her life. This incident further fed her worries and internal imagery, and a vicious cycle was off and running.

Besides using concentration techniques that we discussed in Step 3 to change Beth's prerace focus, I taught her to alter her inner movies to help her get back in control. Through the nightly practice of mental rehearsal, Beth vividly experienced herself remaining happy, composed, and properly focused before her 200. As a consequence of these experiences, Beth was able to stay relaxed before her race. Feeling calmer, her confidence began to return along with feelings of being back in control. (This is a good example of the interconnectedness of the slump-busting model. Concentration and imagery interventions affect feelings of control, confidence, and the ability to handle pressure, all discussed in the model's separate steps.) Soon Beth started to swim fast again without having to leave her lunch on the pool deck.

Correct mental practice can help you restore your shaky confidence and build the positive expectations in your performance that we discussed in the last step. Further, the right kind of mental rehearsal can actually help program your muscles so that they don't abandon you at crunch time. Your imagery practice can then become an integral part of your slump insurance, which we discuss in Step 10. If you can learn to consistently see what you want to happen in your mind's eye, soon everyone watching on the outside will see the same performance played out before them.

Developing Slump-Busting Imagery

It's not unusual for your specific performance difficulty to be represented in your internal imagery. The skater who is stuck on a double axel can't seem to *feel* the jump, and this lack of kinesthetic awareness is reflected in her imagery. She only sees pictures; she can't feel the jump in her mental rehearsal. The ballplayer struggling with throwing problems always sees himself tossing the ball in the dirt or overthrowing first when he attempts his mental rehearsal. He can't see an accurate throw. The high jumper who consistently mistimes her steps and almost runs into the bar can't see anything when she tries to mentally rehearse the correct timing and form. She closes her eyes to imagine and sees nothing but a black slate.

By learning to systematically change different facets of your internal imagery, you can begin to weaken the slump's hold over you. Developing slump-busting imagery takes patience and practice. Whether your images are inaccurate, missing, or the exact opposite of what you'd like, you can still learn to master the skill of mental rehearsal. When perfected, this skill will take you beyond slump-busting to peak performance. The guidelines that follow will help you correctly begin this process and make your slump ancient history.

Check the Accuracy of Your Images

To use mental rehearsal as an internal smart bomb aimed at the performance problem, you need to be clear about what the target is and where it's located. For example, when I used to teach tennis professionally, I knew a player with mechanically deficient strokes. He was quite serious about learning the game, however, and his mind-set was that if you want to do something right, do it yourself. He believed that all anyone really needed was determination and persistence. Every day, all summer long, he'd spend four to six hours stroking the ball the wrong way. With all that practice, his game improved, but was severely handicapped by his faulty stroke mechanics. When I suggested that he would be much better off investing in some lessons to correct his stroke, he politely refused, explaining that he had his own "special" way that worked just fine.

What this player didn't understand was that he was getting better at doing things wrong. He was further ingraining a bad habit. You can't break a bad habit or correct a problem by blindly practicing longer or harder. The only way to really change a faulty technique is to first develop an awareness of what you are doing wrong and then learn how to do it right. Practice does not make perfect; only "perfect practice" does.

Practice does not make perfect; only perfect practice does.

Similarly, if your internal imagery is inadvertently maintaining or contributing to your performance problems, change must start with awareness. As we discussed in the exercise called "What Mental Strategies Are You Using?" in Step 2 (page 28), you have to *recognize* the inner pictures that you're creating now and determine whether these are contributing to or helping you solve the problem. Practicing the wrong mental mechanics will have the same effect as practicing the wrong physical mechanics. They will simply prolong the performance problems. So before you start mentally rehearsing the "correct" strokes, mechanics, or techniques, be sure that what you practice is indeed correct.

How do you know if what you are practicing in your mind's eye is correct? Consult with a trusted outside observer. Ask your coach to help you check the accuracy of your internal images. First, take some time at home to slowly and carefully rehearse your performance. Mentally experience yourself going through your entire performance, paying close attention to the part where you are experiencing difficulty. As you do this or afterward, write down in as much detail as possible all the elements that you must perform for correct execution. What should you be doing with your hands, arms, body position, movement, and so on? How should the movements feel as you go through them? You may have to mentally rehearse your performance several times before you can develop a detailed description of it as you think it should be. Once you've done this, bring your detailed written account to a trusted advisor to check the accuracy of your images. Mentally practicing the wrong things will only contribute to your rut.

As a coach, assigning mental rehearsal as homework to your athletes will help weaken the slump's hold. However, *before* you do this, carefully check the athletes' technical and mechanical grasp of the movements that are giving them trouble. Then have them go through the above exercise of detailing their performance and recording it for you, so that you can check the accuracy of their images. This exercise may also provide you with important clues to their performance problem. Let me explain.

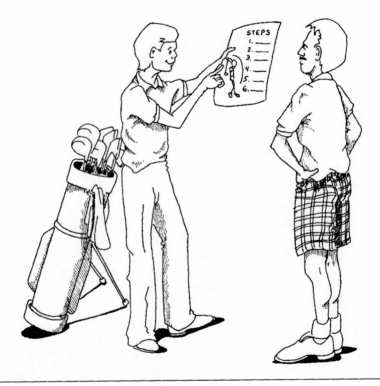

Check the accuracy of your images.

Occasionally, simply analyzing their mental images of their performance will be enough to free athletes from their performance rut. As they systematically think about their performance, they may discover that they were leaving out an important movement or element. This discovery may be all that's needed to interrupt the slump cycle. For example, Latasha was a teenage high jumper who had been stuck at five feet for almost a year and a half. When I first had her check the accuracy of her images for mental rehearsal practice by writing down all the steps that go into her jumps, she suddenly realized that she had been omitting a subtle but important hip movement. She knew that she was supposed to move her hips in this way but hadn't ever seen herself doing it. When she imagined herself going through the jump, she discovered that it was missing. That night she mentally practiced the jump 28 times, concentrating on *seeing* and *feeling* her hips do their thing. The next afternoon in practice, she cleared five feet, two inches!

As you attempt your mental rehearsal, what happens if you can't see or feel anything? You try to turn on the VCR in your mind's eye and the tape jams. Now what? If this happens, just relax and think yourself through the performance anyway, in the proper order. Images or not, write down the steps that you think should be happening. Don't be concerned that you're sitting in the theater and they forgot to turn on the projector.

Once you get assurance from your coach that your understanding of the movements and mechanics are accurate, then you are ready for the next guideline for successful mental rehearsal—your vantage point for these inner movies. Should you view them from inside or outside the action?

Pick the Proper Perspective

You can practice mental rehearsal from a number of perspectives. You can be *outside* the experience looking in or *inside* the experience as if you were actually going through the motions, or you can combine these two. A hammer thrower who was having trouble handling the pressure of big meets exemplifies the *external* perspective. In her mental rehearsals, she always saw herself throwing *as if she were in the bleachers*, watching herself from afar. This perspective helped her consistently practice seeing herself remain composed and calm while competing. A swimmer mentally rehearsing for the 1996 Olympic Trials illustrates the *internal* perspective. Every night for three months, he practiced seeing, feeling, and hearing himself performing *as if he were actually right there* at the competition. A striker for the U.S. National Team mentally practiced taking penalty kicks in pressure situations, using a combination of these two perspectives. She would see herself going for the kick and scoring as if she were watching from the sidelines (external imagery), but *while* she was doing that, she'd actually *feel* herself going through the movements of kicking *as if she were in the action* (internal imagery).

Which method of mental rehearsal will help you most in busting that slump? The answer depends on you as an individual and the nature of your performance difficulty. For example, if one of the primary causes of your slump is a lack of kinesthetic awareness, then it is critical that you learn to develop an *in-the-experience* feeling when you mentally rehearse. Like Latasha, the high jumper, you'll occasionally find that an *outside-the-experience* perspective can provide valuable clues to your performance difficulties. As a general rule, you can benefit from learning how to mentally practice from *both* perspectives. However, mental rehearsal from *inside the experience* is a valuable tool for both preparing for peak performance *and* slump busting.

> *M*ental rehearsal from inside the experience is a valuable tool for preparing for peak performance and slump busting.

The reason for the effectiveness of the inside perspective lies in the critical importance of timing and feel to proper execution in sports. In every sport, having the "right touch" is a prerequisite for peak performance. Kicking a ball, shooting a 15-foot jump shot, smashing an overhead, nailing a flip-turn, and executing a reverse-and-a-half off the three-meter board all require precise timing and feel. Your kinesthetic awareness—your "muscle memory"—helps you repeat these important movements over and over again, regardless of the situation. Consequently, being *inside* the action when you mentally rehearse so that you practice *feeling* the correct mechanics, timing, and execution can be an effective slump-busting technique.

Mentally Rehearse in Vivid Detail

The effectiveness of your mental practice depends largely on your ability to re-create experience in your mind's eye in vivid detail. Try to involve all your senses to see, hear, feel, and even smell the experience. The more lifelike your images, the more powerful they will be in enhancing your performance. A national-caliber roller skater demonstrates this vivid re-creation of experience in how she prepares for a regional qualifying competition. In her nightly imagery sessions leading up to the contest, she *sees* the rink moving around her as she skates in the experience, noticing blurred faces, colors of the advertising banners, and the light reflecting off the shiny wood surface of the rink. As she mentally skates, she can *feel* the power in her legs, the takeoff on her jumps, the in-air rotations of her body, and the cleanness of her landings. Through these mental sessions, she can *hear* the sound of her wheels on the wood surface and the response of the crowd when she nails her tough jumps. She has even developed her imagery to the point where she can *smell* the popcorn from the refreshment stand!

> **T**he more lifelike your images, the more powerful they will be in enhancing your performance.

As you practice mental rehearsal, systematically add sights, sounds, and feelings to your picture. If any of these dimensions are missing for you, try the following progression. Let's say, for example, that you are unable to feel yourself swinging smoothly and powerfully at the plate. Go through the actual physical motions of batting. First, grab your bat and take two or three perfect swings, paying close attention to the feelings in your hands, arms, and body as you do this. Next, sit down, close your eyes, and try to feel the same bat stroke without any movement. If you are still unable to feel anything, continue to alternate this physical and mental practice. With persistence and patience, you will soon begin to feel yourself swinging in your imagery.

If you participate in a sport where you can't easily repeat the proper physical motions in the privacy of your room, set aside a few minutes of practice time to physically break down the activity into its component movements. For example, if you are a swimmer, physically repeat your start, strokes, and turn several times in the pool. Then sit on the pool deck with your eyes closed and try to recapture the kinesthetic feelings of each of these movements. Continue to alternate the execution of the actual movements with the feeling-focused mental rehearsal until you're able to mentally feel the motions.

Use a similar technique with any sense that you're having trouble mentally rehearsing. If your imagery screen is blank when you attempt to mentally practice, no need to panic. Simply alternate physically viewing something with mentally viewing it. For example, if you are a tennis player, you can stand behind the baseline and carefully look out over the court. After taking in this visual information, close your eyes and try to repeat in your mind's eye exactly what you saw. To make this visual practice easier, first look at a tennis ball or racket, and then close your eyes and try to repeat the image. The more difficulty you experience in creating mental imagery, the more you need to practice alternating the actual seeing with the mental seeing.

Ronald was a former four-handicap golfer with rapidly rising scores and frustration. He had been playing golf for 35 years and had developed such a nasty case of the "yips" that he was ready to quit. The yips are golf's version of choking. The golfer gets so nervous over the ball and preoccupied with the outcome that his muscles tighten up and become virtually nonfunctional. Swinging a club with the yips is like trying to run fast under water. While the yips can strike a golfer's swing anywhere on the course, they most frequently attach themselves to the hapless athlete's putting. Putting is the stroke in golf that is the easiest to execute physically yet the hardest mentally. There is more outcome pressure when you're over the ball on the green than any other place on the course. While you may be able to drive the ball 250 yards with only one stroke, getting the ball to travel 20 feet on a green and drop into an impossibly small hole could cost you three strokes *and* your sanity.

Before calling me, Ronald had exhausted every possible avenue of escape from his slump. He had taken putting lessons from *six* different teaching professionals. He had changed his putter *five* times. He had altered his grip, stance, and stroke, all to no avail. Out of desperation, he had even tried putting left handed (he was right handed); but no matter what he tried, he couldn't shake the yips.

Ronald seemed "allergic" to the short grass on the green. First, he'd stand over each putt long enough to hyperventilate. Then as he began the forward part of his stroke, both his wrists would bend to the left, causing him to double hit the ball. It was a mechanically inept stroke and terrifically ugly to watch. Ronald knew that he was supposed to keep his wrists locked and use his arms to stroke the ball. He'd even repeat his latest pro's instructions to himself like a mantra while he was over the ball. However, nothing could change Ronald's wrists from flapping around on the stroke. The wrist snap, which caused the putter head to move sharply to the left, sent all of Ronald's putts way off target and drove him to distraction.

While Ronald could demonstrate the correct locked-wrists form for putting while on the rug in my office, his wrists seemed to have a mind of their own whenever he stood over a ball on the green. What I discovered through the course of our work was that Ronald really had no awareness of what his wrists were actually doing *while* he putted. Intellectually, he knew what they were *supposed* to do. He could even mentally see himself stroking the ball the right way. However, when he was over the ball and putting, he literally could not *feel* his wrists breaking.

When I first had Ronald mentally rehearse the correct stroke, I was confused by his ease at coming up with the proper images. He could see his wrists correctly going through the motion of the stroke without breaking, as if he were actually over the ball. He could even see himself putting correctly as if he were standing on the edge of the green watching himself. However, despite all this successful mental practice, his putting stroke was still a disaster. Something else was going on that was short-circuiting his ability to see the correct stroke.

The cause of the problem and target of our work was Ronald's feel of the stroke. In golf and in most other sports, the proper feel is critical to effective execution. If you can't feel what you're doing, you won't be able to do it right. This is frequently the case for slumping athletes. Because of the distractions going on in their heads, struggling athletes lose the proper feel. Golfers must have "soft hands" to putt well. They must have a certain feeling of relaxation in their fingers, hands, and arms as they stroke the ball. This feel was completely missing for Ronald. When he practiced mental rehearsal, he was oblivious to these feelings. His lack of kinesthetic awareness was consistent with his problem on the green. While Ronald repeated to himself over and over again "keep your wrists locked," he was actually distracting himself from having the proper feeling as he putted.

I asked Ronald to demonstrate for me what the perfect putting stroke would *feel* like. I had him close his eyes and completely focus on the kinesthetic sensations in his hands and arms. When he was able to identify that just-right feeling in his body, I asked him to memorize it. I then had him close his eyes and see if he could *mentally* repeat that same stroke, *concentrating on the proper feel.* I wanted him to understand that the *target of his mental practice was that just-right feel.* As homework I had him mentally rehearse the proper stroke feeling at least 30 to 40 times a day. With this inner practice and a slight adjustment of his over-the-ball concentration, Ronald began to stroke the ball smoothly again; and shortly after that, his yips went away.

For some sports, certain senses are more important than others. For example, when a gymnast or diver executes a skill, a kinesthetic sense or feeling of the movement is absolutely critical. However, the visual imagery of what the gymnast or diver sees during this execution may be a mere blur. It may be only at the end of the trick or dive that the visual becomes important again, as the athlete picks a spot to focus on as a cue to come out of the spin or rotation. Consequently, when the gymnast or diver mentally rehearses, visualizing the move may be slightly less important than feeling the kinesthetics of the move.

Begin Your Mental Rehearsal With Relaxation

So how and when should you practice your slump-busting mental rehearsal? When you're first learning the skill, find a quiet place that is free from distractions. Practicing imagery right before bedtime is frequently ideal. Before you turn on that VCR in your mind's eye, be sure to relax. Mental rehearsal of any kind is more effective when it's preceded by brief periods of relaxation. It doesn't matter what relaxation technique you use before your sessions. All that matters is that you spend a few minutes slowing yourself down and turning your attention inward. Slow, deep breathing is an easy and quick way to calm yourself and get the mental rehearsal working. Progressive muscle relaxation and autogenic training (see the appen-

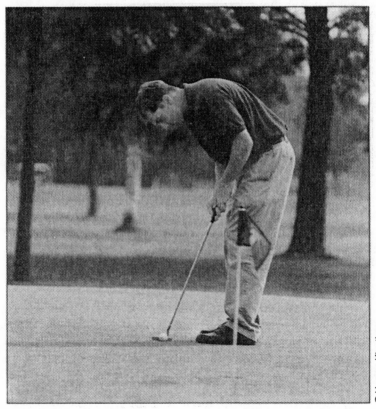

© Human Kinetics

dix for instructions) are also useful relaxation techniques. If you're distracted or anxious before you mentally rehearse, you will be unable to call up useful imagery. Anxiety or stress disrupts visualization, whereas deep relaxation facilitates it. A relaxation script is included at the end of this chapter to guide you.

Keep Your Mental Rehearsal Frequent and Brief

Mental rehearsal works best if you practice frequently for short amounts of time. Five minutes of relaxation followed by five minutes of imagery practice nightly will be more effective than a longer session just once a week. If you spend 20 or more minutes practicing mental rehearsal, your attention will likely drift or you will fall asleep. If you do begin snoring in the middle of your imagery sessions, you may need to change the time of day that you practice or the length of your sessions. Falling asleep is great for restoring your energy and giving your body a chance to recover, but it doesn't do anything for mental rehearsal.

Have a Specific Target for Your Mental Rehearsal

Your imagery sessions will be more effective if you develop a *specific goal* for them. Don't just close your eyes and imagine yourself having an Olympic-caliber performance. While that may excite you, it may not be what you need to break the slump. Instead, your mental rehearsal should have a specific and important target. For example, part of your performance difficulty may be related to your excessive nervousness before a performance. In your imagery sessions, you can practice experiencing yourself remaining calm and composed before the competition and then performing to your potential. The main emphasis here, however, is on maintaining those feelings of relaxation. Similarly, another part of your slump may be fueled by the impact the crowd or the opposing team's comments have on you. You can target your imagery practice at staying centered and focused while the crowd and your opponents are trying to upset you. In your mental rehearsal, you practice tunnel vision to tune out the crowd and the opponents.

Try to pinpoint your performance difficulty and work on correcting it in your mind's eye.

Ask for your coach's assessment of your performance problems, and then target your mental rehearsals at those causes. If your coach thinks that your hands are too tight when you step to the plate, practice feeling soft hands as you take your swings in the on-deck circle and batter's box. If your coach points out that you're bringing your racket head up too high on the backswing, practice seeing and feeling the racket head low when you mentally practice. Try to pinpoint your performance difficulty and work on correcting it in your mind's eye.

Anticipate Problems and Be Persistent

Mental rehearsal is a skill and, like any skill, mastery does not happen overnight. To become proficient takes patience and ample practice. As you attempt to use mental rehearsal as a slump-busting tool, you may experience some problems. You may not be able to see anything, or your images may turn nasty right before your eyes. Keep in mind that this difficulty is expected and does not mean that you cannot effectively use mental rehearsal. Let's take the issue of controllability as an example.

Many athletes first try mental rehearsal because they've heard about how powerful this technique can be in enhancing performance and preparing for an upcoming competition. Having never tried it before, they anxiously look forward to practicing for the big game. When they close their eyes hoping to see themselves throwing the winning touchdown or stopping their opponent's last attempt to score, they are unsettled to see just the opposite happening. They throw an interception. Their opponent kicks the ball by their outstretched arms to score. They hurriedly erase this nightmare and try it a second time. Unfortunately, the next viewing is no different from the first, humiliation and failure. Most athletes at this point think that they would have to have a screw loose to practice seeing themselves fail over and over again, so they give up on mental rehearsal, wrongly thinking that it's not right for them or just doesn't work.

Like every aspect of mental rehearsal, learning to control the images so that you see what you want to happen and not what you're afraid will happen takes time and practice. It is quite natural in the beginning to not have complete control over the images and have them pop up negative. If this happens to you, simply relax and hit the "stop" button on the VCR in your mind's eye and replay the picture. If it comes up negative a second or third time, continue to interrupt the picture and replay it. You may have to slow the picture down and run it in slow motion before you can get the images correct. With enough practice, your imagery sessions will become more productive and will no longer depict failing performance.

Seeing Your Way Out of the Slump

Now that you have a general idea of what mental rehearsal is and some guidelines to make your practice sessions effective, it's time to refine some rehearsal techniques that will take you back to peak performance. The following two imagery exercises will provide some powerful and effective weapons in your fight to break out of your performance doldrums. The first of these, *coping imagery*, is a technique in which you anticipate and systematically prepare for distractions that have previously knocked you off-balance. The second, *mastery imagery*, is a way to practice and ingrain an optimal performance. With regular practice, both of these exercises will help you not only bust that slump, but also build a strong foundation of mental toughness. Both can be used quite effectively in-season as well as off-season.

Coping Imagery

In the coping-imagery technique, the athlete mentally practices encountering stressful or upsetting situations in competition and responding to these upsets in a new, performance-enhancing way. By gaining this experience successfully managing these obstacles, the athlete is better able to cope with them when they arise in actual competition.

To get coping imagery to work for you, first make a detailed list of all the situations that push your emotional hot buttons and cause you to lose control. Your hot buttons can be anything: making mistakes, seeing a particular opponent, getting a bad call from an official, failing, playing in bad weather, hearing boos from the crowd, or receiving an insensitive comment from a coach. Write down each situation that sends your performance into a nosedive. Next, think about an ideal coping response or two for each situation. That is, what would be the perfect way to respond to this particular hot button? Your ideal coping response may involve more than one set of behaviors. For example, if mistakes send you off the deep end, an ideal coping response may include slowing and deepening your breathing or positive self-talk, such as "OK, no problem. Let it go; you'll get it back. Stay in the now and refocus on the contest."

Once you've developed one or more ideal coping responses, mentally practice using them when you're confronted with the stressful hot button situation. Close your eyes, allow yourself to completely relax, and then practice successfully handling the situation by using the coping behavior you picked out. It's useful to follow the coping response with imagery in which you perform flawlessly until confronted with the next stressor. A coping imagery sample script is included for your reference at the end of this chapter.

Coping imagery can help you interrupt the negative, self-maintaining cycle that is the slump. By short-circuiting your slump-feeding, negative emotional reactions with ideal coping responses, you can respond to those old stressors in a more performance-enhancing way. The tape recording that you make to help you mentally practice your ideal coping responses (see the coping imagery sample script at the end of this chapter) will serve as your own personal slump-busting tape. Use this tape and the coping imagery as often as you can to successfully program your new reactions into your internal computer.

> *By short-circuiting your slump-feeding emotional reactions with ideal coping responses, you can respond to those old stressors in a more performance-enhancing way.*

However, a word of caution here. Do not practice coping imagery close to actual competition. If you're in a sport where the competitions are spaced weeks apart, stop using your coping tape about a week before your performance and instead practice mastery imagery, which I'll discuss in the next section. The reason for this is simple. With coping imagery, you are frequently seeing, hearing, and feeling things going less than optimally. While you're practicing quickly rebounding from these bad breaks, errors, or miscues, nevertheless these images are negative. Because your internal imagery has such a powerful impact on programming your performance, it's critical to have only positive, success-oriented imagery in your head as your competition approaches. Consequently, one of the best times to practice coping imagery is during the off-season.

However, once your season starts, if your competitions are spaced only days apart, coping imagery can still be quite useful. Practice the coping imagery at least once between contests, but spend more time with the mastery imagery. When you do use coping imagery with competition close by, be sure to emphasize the recovering quickly, staying in control, peak performance aspects of the imagery.

Mastery Imagery

When you're in the zone and in a peak performance, the world is a wonderful place. Your timing is flawless. Your movements are smooth, powerful, and effortless. You are the perfect balance of mind and body, truly enjoying the beauty of the experience as time seems to stand still. You feel that nothing can interrupt this harmony and knock you off center. World champion Russian weightlifter Yuri Vlasov once described this peak performance experience as "the white moment" and went on to add, "There is no more precious moment in life than this and you will work very hard for years just to taste it again."

While the perfect performance is what all serious and not-so-serious athletes continually strive for, Vlasov's white moment is actually quite elusive. Although you may not be able to walk on water athletically every day, you and your performance problems can still benefit from *pretending* that you can. By regularly practicing mastery imagery—imagining a peak performance—you can break the slump cycle. These positive images will offset the negativity that regularly feeds the slump and will help positively reprogram you to benefit from seeing what you want to happen. Over many years, 1988 Olympic figure skating gold medalist Brian Boitano claimed to have skated the perfect program in his head over a million times before he actually did just that to win the Olympics. Boitano received several perfect 10s from the judges for his final long program that clinched the gold.

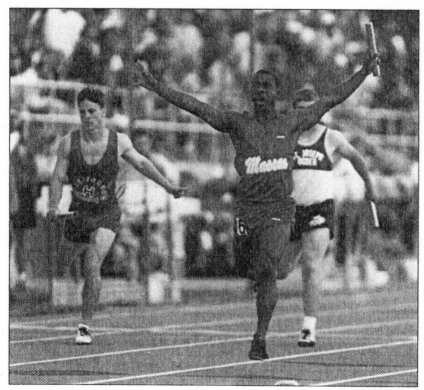

© Human Kinetics

***B**y regularly imagining a perfect performance,
you can break the slump cycle.*

Mastery imagery can help you increase your self-confidence, bust out of that slump mentality, and begin to expect success again. Like coping imagery, this skill should be learned and practiced following the imagery guidelines previously discussed. Similarly, writing a mastery script (see the end of this chapter), recording it, and using the tape to guide your imagery practice sessions is the ideal way to gain the most benefit. You can tape the mastery exercise directly or adapt it to fit your sport and situation.

Developing your own personalized versions of the coping and mastery scripts at the end of this chapter and then setting them to tape will insure that you get the most out of your imagery practice. You can add special touches to your tapes, like favorite songs or the repetition of positive affirmations throughout. You can even set the tape to music, selecting appropriate songs for each segment. For example, during the relaxation phase of the imagery, you can use soothing music or nature sounds (like ocean

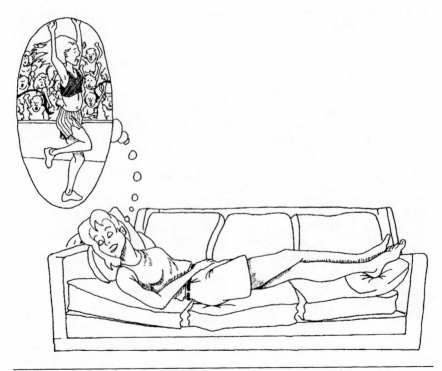

Mastery imagery.

waves or running water) in the background. As you begin to "make friends" with the competitive environment, you can shift the music to a more up-beat tune. As the performance begins, you may shift it once again and continue to do so right through to the celebration at the end of the tape. Personalizing your mastery and coping tapes in this way will make it easier for you to emotionally get into the imagery session.

A final note about imagery practice for coaches and athletes. Some individuals can use mental rehearsal successfully right up until the actual start of their performance. For these athletes, this mental practice becomes part of the preperformance ritual and helps them perform their best. However, many other athletes get too nervous imagining their performance just before the start. Instead, these athletes need to avoid thinking about the upcoming performance in order to be at their best. Mental rehearsal may work very well for these athletes, but only if they do it several hours or days before the competition. How do you determine *when* you should use mental rehearsal? Mainly through trial and error. In the "What Mental Strategies Are You Using?" exercise in Step 2 (pages 27-28), what did you determine that you normally think about before your good and bad performances? Do you do your best when you're *not* thinking about the performance or when you are mentally reviewing it? For example, if your bad performances are preceded by too much performance-related thinking, then mental rehearsal just before the start may not work for you. Instead, try mental rehearsal the days leading up to the performance and don't use it on game day.

This difference among athletes is important for coaches to understand. Many coaches, wanting to integrate mental-toughness training into their programs, insist that *everyone* use mental rehearsal right before the game. This is an unfortunate mistake. As a coach, you should be sensitive to individual differences in your athletes, because what may help prepare one athlete for peak performance may hinder another. In Step 10, "Insuring Against Future Slumps," we will discuss in more depth the topic of individual differences in preperformance preparation.

Conclusion

Because your inner movies have such a profound effect on your performance, it is critical that you learn to take control of what "feature films" you're playing. Slumps are always fueled by the wrong kind of imagery. By following the guidelines discussed in this step and with consistent practice, you can learn to control what you see inside so that you get what you want to happen instead of what you are afraid will happen.

Regular use of mental rehearsal, with or without mastery or coping tapes, will help you permanently shift your thinking away from the slump and toward peak performance. Also, your imagery practice will help you renew your faith in yourself, get back in control, build confidence, and expect success. As a slump-busting tool, developing positive images is directly tied into and positively affects almost every step of the model. As your inner images change, you'll begin to believe in yourself once more, and you can take your dreams and goals off the back burner where they've been sitting all this time because of the slump. As your goals become more believable, your motivation will increase, and the slump will be history.

In the next step in our model, we will focus on the goal-setting process. You will learn how to harness the power of goals to build on the slump-busting momentum that you started when you first picked up this book. By understanding how to use goals effectively, you will have one more weapon in your fight against the slump and a powerful tool for developing mental toughness.

RELAXATION SCRIPT

The best way to use this script is to record it yourself, speaking softly and slowly, pausing for 2 to 3 seconds where indicated by a series of dots (. . .), and then let the tape guide you through the relaxation process. When playing the tape, sit comfortably or lie down in a quiet place where you'll be undisturbed for 10 to 15 minutes. When first learning relaxation, allow for longer sessions (15 to 25 minutes) than you normally would when practicing mental rehearsal (3 to 5 minutes).

Gently close your eyes . . . and focus on your breathing. . . . Slowly follow your breath in . . . and out . . . in . . . and out. . . . Distracting thoughts, like your breath . . . come and go . . . as if an exhaust pipe . . . connects your lungs to your brain . . . and negative thoughts . . . can be exhaled away . . . breathing comfortably in . . . and out. . . . And as you breathe comfortably . . . and begin to relax . . . you let go of the day's tensions. . . .

Remember previous times . . . when you felt relaxed. . . . Remember your own comfortable way . . . of focusing inward . . . and slowing down. . . . And as you follow these words . . . you calm down. . . . You may use them . . . to create your own meaning . . . relaxing the way you'd like. . . . You breathe in comfortably . . . and out . . . in . . . and out. . . . Focus on your breathing . . . and as you do . . . know that your breath has two parts . . . inhalation . . . and exhalation. . . . You take air in . . . and you let it out. . . . You may create an image . . . to link with your breathing. . . .

Some people think about waves . . . as they breathe comfortably in . . . and out. . . . Imagine as you inhale . . . a wave flowing in . . . and breaking on shore . . . and as you exhale . . . the wave slowly recedes. . . . You breathe in . . . and the waves roll in . . . . You breathe out . . . and the waves flow out. . . . When the waves flow in . . . they bring in fresh oxygen. . . . When they flow out . . . they remove carbon dioxide. . . . So too does your breathing . . . inhale energy into your body . . . and exhale fatigue. . . .

You breathe in relaxation. . . . You breathe out tension and negativity. . . . Feel your breathing relax . . . different parts of your body . . . as your breath bathes them. . . . As you watch the waves . . . slowly come in . . . and slowly go out . . . your images may be clear . . . or foggy. . . . You may see boats . . . or beach grass . . . or the sand. . . . You may even hear . . . familiar sounds . . . as the waves come in . . . and go out. . . . You may hear the waves breaking . . . and receding. . . . You may see the sun . . . peeking from behind a cloud . . . slowly warming your body. . . .

You can feel a warmth . . . slowly move over your body. . . . It may start at your fingertips . . . and move up from there . . . or start in your face . . . or in your stomach . . . and move down from there. . . . Feel that warmth and relaxation now. . . . Let yourself go however you'd like . . . as you comfortably inhale . . . and slowly exhale. . . .

And as you relax more . . . you may play in the waves . . . . You may feel the water . . . around your body . . . and imagine with each new breath . . . the waves get smaller. . . . You breathe in . . . and the wave flows in . . . a little smaller than before. . . . You breathe out. . . . You breathe in . . . and the waves get smaller . . . and smaller and smaller . . . and soon the water calms down . . . and appears very still. . . . The water flattens . . . until the surface is completely calm . . . like the surface of a reflecting pool . . . when there's no hint of breeze . . . calm and quiet . . . relaxing more and more . . . breathing in . . . and out . . . feeling relaxed all over. . . .

COPING IMAGERY SEQUENCE

In this example, imagine you are a college softball player whose hitting has been slumping. Your hot buttons are having to hit when there are runners on base, striking out, or otherwise coming up empty in an at-bat. In the past when confronted with these situations, you'd get down on yourself and become angry—swearing, throwing your batting helmet, and punching the dugout walls. Your ideal coping response to having to hit with runners on is to (1) tell yourself to relax and slow down, (2) trust yourself and just let it happen, (3) breathe slowly and calmly, (4) narrow your concentration on the feeling of soft hands, and (5) watch the ball in the pitcher's hand.

You can learn to use coping imagery most effectively by writing a detailed script of the performance and then talking this script slowly into a tape recorder. Then play the tape as a guide each time you practice coping imagery. Your script should include several scenarios in which you are confronted by your stressors and respond by successfully using your ideal coping responses. To increase its effectiveness, your script should begin with a few minutes of relaxation. Use the preceding relaxation script and the sample coping script below as guides to help you develop and personalize your own coping tape.

As in the relaxation exercise, a series of dots (. . .) in the scene below indicates a 2 to 3 second pause.

You've been looking forward to this game all day. You're feeling comfortable. It feels good to warm up. You really like playing in front of the home crowd. You sneak a peek into the stands and find some familiar faces. As you make eye contact with them, it feels good to see their smiles in return. You bring yourself back to the warm-up. Your throws feel clean, smooth, and crisp. You can hear the pop of the ball in the gloves as you play catch. You feel loose and relaxed. Your mind is quiet and you know that you're ready. It's a perfect day to play this team. The sun is warm and there's barely a breeze. You breathe deeply and comfortably as you tell yourself, "Trust yourself; you're ready. . . . Just have fun and let it happen."

You hear the coach yell something about time for batting practice. . . . For a moment you get a twinge of nervousness as you head over to take your cuts. There's that old voice of self-doubt trying to talk to you about your hitting slump, when you suddenly find yourself taking control. "Relax. . . . You can do it. . . . Just stay loose and trust yourself. . . . Let it happen. . . . Stay focused. . . . Breathe comfortably and deeply." . . . And then you do. . . . You're starting to relax more and get back in control. . . . You're beginning to feel stronger as you step up to take your cuts. You remember to feel soft hands as you concentrate your attention on that easy feeling. As you watch the ball coming in, you can see it clearly. Your first swing is a good one. You immediately get that solid feeling as you hear the sweet ping of the ball against the bat. You watch the ball heading deep into the outfield. You hear your teammates yell their approval. . . . You feel confident and in control.

A few pitches later, you foul-tip three balls in a row . . . and then dribble two more back to the pitcher. You begin to hear that little voice of self-doubt creeping up again. . . . That unsettled feeling just starts rising in the pit of your stomach, when you hear yourself taking control. . . . "Relax now. . . . Forget those doubts. . . . Stay loose and trust yourself. . . . Let it happen. . . . You can do it.". . . You breathe slowly and deeply. . . . Then you shift your concentration to feeling those soft hands. . . . You tell yourself again to just relax and watch the ball . . . nice and easy. The next two pitches come in and you crush each of them. . . . You're feeling back in control. . . . You're feeling strong and powerful. . . . Bring on the other team. . . . You're ready now. . . . Let's get this show on the road. . . .

As the game starts, you're feeling pretty good. . . . You're loose and focused. . . . In the field things are easy and effortless. The only ball that's hit to your position, you field cleanly, easily nailing the runner for the out. When the sides are retired, you sprint back to the dugout, ready to hit. You sit on the bench and breathe slowly and comfortably. . . . You tell yourself, "Stay calm and loose. . . . Trust yourself." You're in control. . . . Your team gets on the opposing pitcher right away. A single is followed by a walk and another single loads the bases. You step into the on-deck circle and look over the infield. The home crowd is getting louder as they anticipate some runs being scored. As you watch the batter get behind in the count, you suddenly think that you may have to hit with the bases loaded. You start feeling that nervous stomach again. Before that other part of you can even finish the negative chatter in your head, you interrupt it by saying to yourself, "Slow down and get back in control. Relax.". . . You take a slow, deep breath and feel yourself calming down. You hear those comforting words again. . . . "Trust yourself. . . . Just let it happen." You tell yourself, "Breathe slowly and deeply. . . . Feel those soft hands.". . . And as you do, you narrow your focus onto the pitcher and the ball. You're back in control.   →

When the batter before you strikes out, you're ready. You confidently step up to the batter's box and move the dirt around the way you usually do. You can feel the looseness in your hands and confidence flowing inside. You dig in and plant your feet. You take a slow, deep breath and narrow your focus on the ball in the pitcher's hand. She looks you straight in the eyes, gets the signal from the catcher, and comes at you with a rising pitch. You take a huge cut, but your swing is too late. You momentarily feel stupid. . . . You wonder if you'll be able to hit her. . . . You briefly flash on your hitting slump. . . . Then you hear that reassuring voice in your head, helping you get back in control. . . . "Slow down and breathe. . . . Take your time. . . . One pitch at a time . . . you can do it. Relax and focus on that ball. . . . Trust and let it happen." The next pitch is just like the first, with a lot of heat on it. This time, however, you're ready and waiting. Your swing is smooth and powerful. Your contact is perfect and solid. The sound of the ball on the bat brings the crowd to their feet. You catch a glimpse of the ball going deep to left-center, right between the two outfielders. . . . You put your head down and run. As you round first and pick up speed, you feel unstoppable. The hit was perfect. You're at full speed as you round second and get the go-ahead from the third base coach. As you close on the bag, you get the signal to slide. You time it just right and slide beautifully under the third baseman's glove, hearing the umpire's "safe" call ringing in your ears. The crowd is going nuts, and as you get up and brush yourself off, you can't help but break into a huge smile. The coach catches your eye and let's you know her approval. Kiss that slump good-bye. . . . You're a winner. . . . You're in control.

Two innings later you come up to the plate with two on and two out. The game is now tied. The crowd applauds you loudly when your name is announced over the loudspeaker. Your coach gives you the "hit away" signal, and as you dig in at the plate, you feel ready and strong. It's clear that the pitcher remembers you, because she starts throwing different stuff. You get behind in the count and feel sure she'll try to blow it by you with another rising pitch. You get set. The count is one ball and two strikes. The pitcher winds up and delivers, surprising you with a change-up and catching you completely off guard. Your swing hits nothing but air. There's a loud groan from the crowd. Strike three. . . . You're out. . . . You start to get disgusted with yourself. . . . Your anger is rising. . . . You start thinking slump again, when like clockwork you step in and establish control. . . . "Slow down. . . . Stay loose. . . . It's OK. . . . Let it go. . . . You'll get it back. . . . Just trust yourself and let it happen. . . . No problem.". . . This self-talk is followed by two or three automatic, slow, deep breaths as you begin to feel more in charge. . . even stronger. . . . You recognize that you can maintain your control. . . . You're feeling mentally tough. . . . It doesn't matter what is thrown at you now. . . . You're beginning to be in complete control. . . . As you sprint onto the field to take your position, you leave the memory of that mistake behind. . . . It's gone . . . in the past, and the next at-bat will be different. . . . But even that thought fades quickly as you warm-up and begin to narrow your focus on the task at hand.

This next inning is like a test that you pass with flying colors. On the first pitch, the batter lines a shot to your left. You react perfectly, diving for the ball and making a spectacular grab. The crowd and your teammates roar their approval. . . . You acknowledge it and feel even stronger and more focused now. "In control" keeps popping into your head. "Trust and let it happen" is your mantra. . . . You're feeling relaxed and intense at the same time. This is who you are as an athlete . . . performing with the excellence that you know is inside you. A walk puts the game-winning run on first, one out. The next batter is strong and hit for extra bases earlier in the game. You're in your usual ready position as the pitch is thrown. Instinctively, you take a small step to the right as the pitcher delivers. The batter takes a big cut and crushes a drive sharply to your right toward the hole. Again you react and dive with glove outstretched, eyes narrowed, as you just barely snag the ball before it could get by you. The runner on first is halfway to second and trying desperately to get back to first, as you get out of your prone position and rifle the ball to first, nailing her by a full step. Three outs; inning over. . . .

You run off the field feeling more and more confident . . . more and more in control. . . . You let yourself soak up the cheers and pats on the back. . . . You're feeling good. You're trusting yourself. . . . You experience a strange conviction that your next at-bat will be a good one. . . . Inside you know you'll get a hit. . . . Your chance comes in the bottom of the first extra inning. The score is tied. A runner is on. There are two outs as you step to the plate. You can almost feel yourself smiling inside at the pitcher. . . . You're calm and confident. You want it to be this way. . . . You're almost surprised at this new "old" feeling. . . . You recognize it as how you used to feel all the time when you played. . . . You always wanted to be there when the game was on the line. You wanted your bat on the ball. . . . And now you're there again. . . . You feel yourself relaxing even more. . . . You hear those

→

comforting words in your head. . . . "Relax and slow down. . . . You're in control. . . . Trust yourself and let it happen . . . effortless effort.". . . You take a slow, deep breath as you dig in at the plate and narrow your focus on the mound and the ball in the pitcher's hand. . . . You remember the change-up that she beat you with last time and confidently know that she won't get away with it this time. . . .

The pitcher winds up and delivers, and the ball has your name on it. You see it clearly, all the way in, time your swing perfectly, and crush it. . . . The ball flies off your bat deep to center, clearing the center fielder's desperately outstretched glove. . . . You bolt to first with the crowd's whoops and hollers echoing in your ears. You make the turn and continue for second, as your teammate crosses home plate to seal the win. You stop at second, and the umpire makes it official. The game is over! . . . You're mobbed by the entire team. . . . Even while you celebrate, you can still hear and feel that new-found control and confidence inside as if it were underlining the new changes that you've made. . . . "Relax and stay loose. . . . You're in control. . . . Trust yourself and just let it happen.". . . You automatically take a slow, deep breath as your teammates are going crazy with celebration all around you. . . . As you exhale, you know you're in control and break out into a huge smile as you join them in yelling and screaming.

MASTERY IMAGERY SEQUENCE

To increase the effectiveness of this and any imagery session, begin with a brief period of relaxation. (Refer back to the relaxation script or to any of the exercises mentioned in the appendix.) If you are taping this script, keep in mind that a series of dots (. . .) indicates a pause of 2 to 3 seconds. It's the pauses throughout the exercise that provide you with enough time to create the images and feelings elicited by the sound of your voice.

How do you as an athlete learn to trust yourself when you perform?. . . Perhaps you have a particular competition in mind that you're preparing for or you may simply be in the process of building your self-confidence. . . . In either case, you can catch yourself moving forward into the future. . . . It's as if you have your own personal time machine. . . . You can adjust the dials . . . and somehow you sense that as you begin to enter the future . . . as if it were right now . . . things have powerfully changed for you. . . . Do you feel mentally tougher? . . . More positive? . . . Have a tenacious, never-say-never attitude? . . . Or perhaps you simply feel more confident. . . . As you emerge into the future right now, you notice a new feeling of comfort and ease within yourself. . . . Perhaps you can feel it in how you walk or in the way you carry yourself. . . . Maybe it's that new sense of trust that you have in yourself. . . . Or maybe you feel that you're just more in control, and no other words can describe it. . . .

You can think about that performance, only hours away. You are reviewing all the steps that you've had to take to get here today . . . the hard training . . . the sacrifice . . . your pursuit of that special goal . . . all the obstacles that you've been able to overcome and put behind you. . . . The slump's in the past. . . gone. . . . You can feel a sense of pride in yourself that all those old problems are so comfortably ancient history right now. . . . You've refused to give up, and your determination has paid off. . . . You can even feel this sense of accomplishment in your breathing . . . in a feeling that you can hold your head up and stand taller. . . .

You become aware of a growing sense that you're ready . . . really ready. . . . You've paid your dues . . . done everything in your power to get here . . . and you can feel good about your training. . . . You feel a sense of comfortable anticipation as you think about this performance and recognize that you're at an energizing level of nervousness . . . those familiar feelings in your body . . . stomach . . . breathing . . . that

→

let you know you're physically and mentally in the right place. . . . It's nice to notice these changes in your body as you get ready to perform and know that they will take you to the level of excellence that's inside you. . . .

And as you come out of these inner thoughts, you look around . . . . You find yourself in the competition arena and it's a few hours before the start. . . . You may be alone or with a trusted teammate or coach . . . but the arena is otherwise silent and empty. . . . Take some quiet time to make friends with the environment . . . one small step at a time . . . . Walk out there and look around. . . . You can quietly and confidently take in all the familiar sights of the sport that you've grown to love and in which you excel. . . . And as you look around, you can imagine where the audience will be . . . the officials . . . your opponents. . . . You begin to feel yourself comfortably in control. . . .

As you feel that growing sense of security, you begin to notice those familiar sounds. . . . Since the competitive arena is empty, many of those sounds are absent for the time being. . . . You can certainly imagine hearing them as you look around . . . and you are pleasantly surprised by the confident voice you can hear inside you, reminding you over and over, "You're ready. . . . You belong here. . . . Trust yourself and let it happen.". . . And as you continue to move around the arena, you know you can handle anything thrown at you. . . . You have had the experience of feeling really confident before, and that confidence propelled you to greatness. . . . "Trust and let it happen."

And as you leave the nearly empty arena, you allow your eyes to take one final look around. . . . You feel calm and ready . . . confident and composed. . . . And as you turn your back to leave, you hear those guiding words again from inside you: "Just trust yourself and let it happen. . . . You're ready . . . trust and let it happen.". . .

Now transport yourself to just a few moments before your competition. . . . Almost everything has changed now since your last trip. . . . The air is electric with excitement and anticipation. . . . You are able to hear a loudspeaker announcing in the background . . . the noise of the crowd . . . other competitors . . . the voice of your coaches or teammates. . . . You briefly look around, calmly taking it all in. . . . You find it interesting that you can feel so composed and confident with all the noise and distractions going on around you. . . . And even with all the noise . . . you still hear the comforting echo of those words in the back of your mind . . . those words that keep you focused and positive, "Trust yourself and let it happen. . . . You're ready. . . .

Trust and let it happen.". . . And as you hear those words, you can recognize a familiar and comfortable looseness within your body. . . . You feel good . . . energized . . . powerful . . . and your muscles feel the way they always do just before you do your very best. . . .

You begin to narrow your concentration as the seconds tick away before the start. . . . And how do you narrow your focus in a championship way just before performance?. . . You can do this by beginning that old, familiar ritual that you always go through . . . that special routine that calms you and helps get you centered . . . you move a certain way . . . stretch a certain way . . . talk to yourself a certain way. . . . You begin to mentally review the upcoming performance and exactly how you'd like it to go today. . . . And it doesn't matter what your ritual is, or whether you call it a routine or superstition, all that matters is that you take the time right now to calmly and confidently go through it. . . . And as you do, in the back of your mind you continue to hear those calming words, like a mantra, soothing you . . . focusing you. . . . "Trust yourself and just let it happen."

Now you narrow your focus by distracting yourself so that there are no thoughts going on in your head. . . . You just blank everything out. . . . You know that you'll do your best when you're on automatic and not thinking. . . . And it really doesn't matter what you do to get yourself ready right before the performance. . . . All that matters is that you are calm and focused . . . confident and ready. . . .

Now you transport yourself to the start. . . . As you see and hear the contest begin, you are pumped and loose at the same time, exploding into action as if you've been down this familiar path many times before. . . . You are aware of a sense of power . . . and at the same time an effortlessness and ease to your movements. . . . It's as if you're already on automatic . . . performing as practiced. . . . Your concentration is so focused that you have tunnel vision. . . . You're an athlete on a mission. . . . The initial butterflies you felt just before the start have been constructively channeled into your performance. . . . Your muscles feel loose and energized. . . . Your technique and mechanics feel flawless, your movements are smooth and efficient. . . . You already know that you're on . . . you're in your zone. . . . But you're not distracted by anything around you . . . just a laserlike focus on the task at hand. . . . You have a deja-vu feeling of having been here many times before. . . . A fleeting thought—your imagery practice sessions have really paid off . . . because here you are, right now, living that dream of the perfect performance. . . .

→

As the event proceeds, your intensity and focus increase. You're performing as planned. . . . You feel strong and have a sense that you could go all day. . . . You keep your mind on the task at hand . . . feeling stronger and more confident. . . . You find it easy to trust yourself. . . . You know that you're in a let-it-happen mentality. . . . Nobody and nothing can stop you, as you continue to move your arms . . . legs . . . and body in those so familiar patterns that you don't even have to think about. . . . You're like a fine-tuned machine. . . . Your timing is flawless . . . your mechanics smooth. . . . You're surprised to notice how much you can enjoy the performance . . . even while the intensity of it flows all around you. . . .

Moving into the middle of the performance, you are approaching a point that previously had created a few problems for you. . . . It is quite interesting how you can move into and through this point smoothly and effortlessly . . . feeling in complete control . . . dominating . . . powerful . . . with no other thoughts except those related to what's going on around you as you move. . . . Opponents, fans, officials, the media all fade into the background . . . as if you know they are uncontrollable and of no value to you . . . so you simply block them out and keep your attention on yourself and what you're doing. . . . Whatever comes your way, you easily and smoothly handle . . . rebounding quickly and refocusing with an added intensity . . . just flowing . . . trusting and letting it happen . . . trusting and letting it happen.

Sooner or later every competition reaches that critical point . . . maybe a deciding point. . . . It could be somewhere in the middle or right near the end . . . a point when every movement takes on added importance. . . . You see yourself moving through this point in the performance now . . . and feel yourself there . . . and you can even recognize certain sounds from around you that let you know it's truly crunch time. . . . You're delighted at how easily you can maintain your concentration and control. . . . The bigger the moment, the more efficient and focused you can get. . . . You still feel loose and smooth . . . totally in control and persevering. . . . You are rising to the challenge and taking your place out in front . . . separating yourself from the competition. . . . You're on a mission, and nothing can get in your way. . . . You push to the finish . . . the end is in sight . . . and it is curious how that fact is way in the back of your mind . . . because even as you know that, your concentration is locked in the here and now where it should be . . . taking it one movement at a time . . . totally oblivious to the outcome. . . .

You now finish that perfect performance. . . . Is it a burst of speed? . . . A series of movements that exhibit perfect feel and timing? . . . One final output of strength and mastery? . . . The images get sharper and brighter as you come to the end. . . . You more clearly hear the roar of the crowd, your teammates, and coaches. . . . You become aware of a rush of feeling that lets you know that you've done it . . . amazingly so. . . . It's over . . . and it was unbelievable . . . just the way you'd envisioned it. . . . You can begin to feel a sense of relief. . . . You've achieved a level of excellence that makes you feel really good about yourself . . . and you sense the appreciation for a job well done . . . a difficult mission finally accomplished. . . .

As you begin to really take in your accomplishment . . . breathing in and out slowly and deeply . . . how do you celebrate? . . . Can you feel yourself smiling? . . . Can you see the joy on the faces of those who support you? . . . Can you feel the high-fives and hugs all around? . . . the back slapping? . . . Are there tears of joy? . . . You can hear those heartfelt congratulations from the people you really care about. . . .

You feel a growing sense of confidence . . . an inner trust in yourself and your abilities . . . a trust that you can take away with you today and use tomorrow and the next day. . . . You slowly take another deep breath . . . allowing the scene to gradually fade . . . and letting your awareness slowly return to this room and this time.

7

SETTING SLUMP-BUSTING GOALS

"Inch by inch anything's a cinch . . .
yard by yard it'll be too hard."

As a serious athlete, you can't reach your true athletic potential without well-conceived, realistic goals. You need a clear picture of where you want to go if you ever hope to get there. Your goals serve as your guide. They both create and illuminate the pathway into the future. They let you know where you are in your personal pursuit of excellence and what you need to successfully finish the journey. Along the way, goals can help you get around the road blocks and through the rough spots that are a normal part of that journey.

If effectively using goals is one of the big secrets to achieving success in and out of sports, why doesn't everyone immediately harness their awesome power? Unfortunately, many athletes either take goal setting for granted or simply don't understand it well enough to use it effectively. Because success is a chance event without proper goals, many athletes end up stuck with "permanent potential" because they misused or ignored the goal-setting process. In fact, a lot of athletes struggle with slumps because they don't understand the why and how of goal setting.

S*uccess is a chance event without proper goals.*

In our description of the principles of peak performance (see the Introduction), we discussed the importance of having a process focus rather than an outcome focus when you perform. Athletes who focus on *what* they are doing *while* they are doing it, a process focus, perform better than those who worry about the competition's outcome, for example, winning, scoring two touchdowns, making the varsity, raising their batting average, qualifying for nationals, and so on. *When* you are performing, your goals represent an outcome or future focus and therefore are an uncontrollable (see Step 2). Since a focus on uncontrollables just *before* and *during* performance will raise your stress, lower your confidence, and set you up to fail, *taking your goals into the competitive arena with you is a slump-fueling mental mistake.*

Rather than unknowingly using your goals to sabotage your performance and feed your slump, learn how to harness the power of goal setting to snap out of your performance doldrums. Our focus for this next step in the slump-busting model is on how to set effective and specific goals to break the slump and build motivation and mental toughness.

Goal setting for slump busting functions like a magnifying glass reflecting sunlight onto a dead branch. When the magnifying glass is held at just the right angle and distance between the sun and the wood, it collects and condenses all the sun's energy into a narrow, powerful beam that scorches the wood. In a similar way, setting and using clear, specific goals when working on your slump will focus your energy to help you "burn through" your performance difficulties and free up your athletic potential.

For example, let's say that your slump is being supported by poor concentration, negative self-talk, and an inability to stay calm under pressure. By attacking these problems using this step's principles of effective goal setting, you can fine-tune your skills of concentration (Step 3), positive self-talk and reframing (Step 5), positive imagery (Step 6), and relaxation (Steps 6 and 10). Soon these newly acquired skills will help you restore your performance to its preslump level.

The Importance of the Goal-Setting Process

Goals function the way a map would if you were planning a road trip. Let's say, for example, that you live in Boston and want to take a trip. You decide to journey cross-country by car to San Francisco, and you want to get there in two weeks. To reach the "city by the bay" on time, you need a *detailed* map for your trip. You need to know every major and minor road you must take along the way from your starting point in Boston until you spy the Golden Gate Bridge leading into San Francisco. You also need a good idea about how much time the entire trip will take, along with the times of the various legs along the way. If you enlist AAA to help you come up with the plan, like an experienced and trusted coach, they can supply all this information.

G*oal setting is the most important planning and evaluation tool in constructing your athletic career.*

Goal setting is probably the most important planning and evaluation tool you can use in constructing your athletic career. When used properly, the goals that you set as an athlete fuel your motivation. If your targets are personally meaningful, they'll help you justify in your own mind the sacrifices, hard work, and pursuit of excellence you've undertaken. In short, goals give you a *reason* for following the peak performance formula of getting comfortable being uncomfortable.

The Road to Success

A question that confronts every serious athlete at one time or another in their training is "why bother?" They think, "Why should I get comfortable with the physical exhaustion and pain; the stress and emotional ups and downs; and the sweating, injuries, boredom, loneliness, and fears that are all necessary to become a champion?" This question becomes even more compelling when your performance is slumping and your confidence is at an all-time low. It would be much easier to become a couch spud. The only reasonable answer to this question is *because I want to become a champion!* The quest and goal have to be important to *you.* If the goal is more meaningful to your parents, coaches, or friends than it is to you, then you will be less motivated to endure the hardships, disappointments, frustration, and sacrifices that are an integral part of the journey.

A way that I approach goal setting with athletes is by asking them, "Do you know what road you're on?" Training in sports toward a distant goal is like being on a long journey. As you travel, the road continually forks, requiring you to decide which way to go (see figure 7.1). Do you take the left fork or the *right* one? These forks represent all the decisions you're constantly faced with as an athlete. "Do I blow my training diet and have that whole chocolate cake?" "Am I really going to put in those extra hours today?" "I've been playing so badly lately, what difference could it make if I skip weight training just this week?" "Should I run as hard as I can in this wind sprint, even though the coach isn't looking?" "Should I worry about getting in shape after the summer?" "Do I stay up past curfew because no one will know if I break it?"

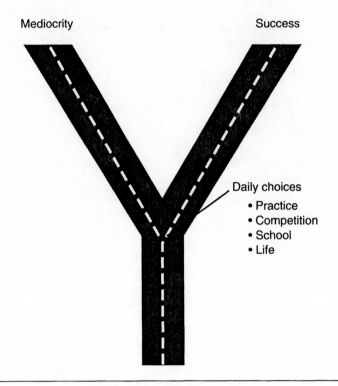

Figure 7.1 Do you know which road you're on?

When you decide in practice to relax when the coach turns his back, you've just made a decision to head down the left fork to mediocrity. When you cheat on the number of laps you say you ran, you've again decided on the road to mediocrity. This road is always the easiest to take, especially when you're in a slump. It requires no special talent. It requires no character. You may briefly fool the coach, but ultimately this path leads to mediocrity. You'll never become a champion by taking the easy road, nor will the easy road lead you out of your performance problems.

> **Y**ou'll never become a champion by taking the easy road, nor will the easy road lead you out of your performance problems.

The other direction, the *right one*, is never as easy to take. This one confronts you with more obstacles, pain, and aggravation. The right fork hurts more. It makes you feel more uncomfortable, both emotionally and physically. Sometimes it makes you cry. However, the right fork, when consistently taken, will always lead you out of the valley of slump to the peak of success. When you decide against going to the movie with your friends and instead spend the time training, you've taken the *right* road. When you push yourself to the limit in each practice, you've headed down that *right* fork. When you get up early and go to practice, even though you really want to stay in bed, you're headed toward success. When you decide to look at your performance problems and weaknesses directly rather than avoid them, you've gone the *right* way.

The Big-Enough Why

Taking the right fork is about living the formula for peak performance: getting comfortable being uncomfortable. There is little discomfort down the road to mediocrity. Therefore, it is critical that you have a goal that will help you make the right choice whenever the road splits in front of you. Your goal has to provide you with enough impetus to do the uncomfortable. To sustain you down this path as a motivational fuel through slumps and hard times, your goal must qualify as a "big-enough why."

This big-enough why is the ultimate dream that keeps you going in the sport. It's that long-range, huge, possibly scary goal. It may be that full college scholarship, making the national team, becoming an Olympian, or playing as a professional. It could be your own personal version of one of these or simply the intense desire to prove yourself. Your big-enough why defines you and uniquely separates you from everyone else. When you keep your big-enough why close to you throughout your training, it will help you stay focused and on track. It will help you put that slump in perspective. When you're physically and emotionally running on empty, ready to quit and head down the road to mediocrity, your big-enough why gives you the guts and determination to keep going the right way. A big-enough why will help you consistently accomplish what all the "experts" tell you is impossible.

> **Y**our big-enough why gives you the determination
> to keep going the right way.

In his book *The Edge*, Howard Ferguson tells the story of Pittsburgh Steeler Rocky Bleier.[1] In 1968, the Pittsburgh Steelers used their last pick in the draft to select Bleier. Unfortunately for Bleier, Uncle Sam also drafted him—for Vietnam. While he was in Vietnam, Bleier had the bottom of his right foot ripped open by a grenade, his right leg shredded by shrapnel, and his left thigh shot up by gunfire. He was listed as 40 percent disabled and sent home.

In 1970, still wanting to play football and unable to even walk without a noticeable limp, Bleier trained for what most considered a futile attempt at a comeback. He got up early to run. In training camp that year, he found himself battling seven healthy running backs for five spots. During the camp, refusing to face reality, Bleier convinced himself that he actually had a chance to make the ballclub. Despite the advice of the experts—coaches, doctors, and trainers—that he should give up football rather than risk more permanent injury, Rocky kept at it. His big-enough why helped him take that right fork again and again. Bleier was the last player cut from the roster that year.

He underwent another foot operation and worked for another shot at the NFL the next season. "I tried to rationalize my workout. Ten laps, two and one half miles. That's all I could do," Bleier remembered. "My right toes ached; I still couldn't push off them. I was still running cockeyed on the heel and side of my foot. My toes had no strength, no endurance, no flexibility. I couldn't do any more." Then Bleier said he would think of the rookies coming in who could effortlessly run 10 laps. He'd imagine he was in super shape, running the football, breaking tackles, the crowd roaring. These images gave him the emotional charge to get up and run more.

Every day when he woke up, with almost every step he took, Bleier was confronted by that fork in the road. Describing his off-season training ritual, Bleier stated, "How can I tell you the agony and tedium of that routine? The physical pain of those mornings—the creaking of my joints and the dull ache of my legs—was matched only by mental anguish of knowing what lay in wait. Something in my head said, 'Go back to sleep. Who's going to know if you miss this one lousy workout?'"

What kept him going against such great odds? At the next training camp, he ripped a hamstring muscle in the leg that had been shot in Vietnam, and instead of listening to the doctors, Bleier taped it up and returned to the field. By 1972 he was playing every game for the Steelers on their special teams. He was timed faster than he had been *before* he suffered his wounds. In 1974, Bleier moved to the starting backfield. In 1976, he gained over 1,000 yards and became one of the key players in Pittsburgh's dominance in the '70s.

Guts and determination stories like Rocky Bleier's are commonplace in the lives of successful people in and out of sports. They are testimony to the get-comfortable-being-uncomfortable formula for goal achievement. They point to the incredible motivational and slump-busting power of a big-enough why. These stories also speak to that superperformer inside us all and the almost unstoppable power of the human spirit when we set our sights on a goal.

When most athletes hit that fork in the road, they abandon the right path. They trade what they want *the most* for what they want *at the moment*. They exchange their dreams for temporary relief and comfort. This kind of exchange is a primary reason why people fail to reach their goals. Taking the harder path is easier if you keep that big-enough why in front of you. By following the principles of winning goal setting found in this step, your efforts and sacrifices to stay on the right road and bust that slump will pay off.

The Principles of Winning Goal Setting

How can you successfully harness all the slump-busting power of goal setting? Simple! Follow the rules. To develop goal-setting skill and get it to work *for* rather than *against* you, use the nine principles of winning goal setting that follow. These nine principles will guide your efforts and channel your energies, so that you will soon be able to replace your subpar performances with those that reflect your true athletic skills and winning attitude.

Principle #1—Be Sure the Goal Is *Yours*

To be successful, you must first be sure that your big-enough why is indeed *yours*. It has to have *your* signature all over it. The goal must have a place in *your* heart. If the goal belongs to someone else, when the going gets tough, you'll ultimately lack the motivation to see it through. Furthermore, if you are training for someone else instead of yourself, performance problems are sure to emerge and continue. Your goal doesn't belong to you if a coach or parent is overly invested in your success and wants the goal more than you do. While having someone push you is important to reaching your goals, this shoving can only work if you *truly* want to be pushed and really desire the prize at the end.

> *T*he goal must have a place in your heart.

For example, Alicia was a 12-year-old, level 9 gymnast with a dream of someday making it to the elite level and possibly to the national team. Her bedroom at home was a testimony to this big-enough why. Her walls were adorned with medals, ribbons, and posters of the Olympic team and her favorite gymnasts. She had gymnasts decorating her bed quilt and gymnasts on her sheets. Trophies from meets were scattered all around the room. Her parents were extremely supportive and offered Alicia every opportunity to pursue *her* goal. As the most talented gymnast in her school, Alicia was a workhorse in the gym. She trained harder than anyone else and was always asking the coaches for more work. When she broke her foot vaulting, she didn't miss one day of practice the four months that she was in a cast. During that time, she found other skills to work on that didn't hurt her foot.

Alicia refused to let anyone or anything get in the way of *her* goal. She got frustrated with teammates who seemed more interested in having a good time than pursuing excellence. She didn't hesitate to express these feelings directly when their behavior interfered with her training. Alicia also felt that the head coach wasn't taking her or her dream very seriously and that he spent too much practice time playing non–performance-related games. When she told him privately that she wanted to work on harder skills, he responded by telling her she was much too serious and needed to have more fun like the other girls.

Alicia became more and more unhappy with the "fun and games" atmosphere in the gym, because she felt like it was a distraction from her goals. After several more frustrating meetings with the coach where she asked for more intensive training and he casually dismissed her requests, Alicia thought about switching gyms. There was a higher-level, more competitive gymnastics school one hour from her house. When she mentioned this move, her coaches responded negatively and told her that such a switch would be a big mistake. They claimed that this other gym pushed their athletes much too hard and really didn't care about them as individuals. The head coach asked Alicia if the idea to change gyms was her mother's, believing that the girl was being pushed into this against her will. Alicia patiently explained once more that *she* was the one who wanted to change gyms because *she* wanted to get more intensive training.

With her parents' permission, Alicia spent two afternoons visiting this new club and working out with their team. There, she was no longer the best athlete in the gym. In fact, she was probably the weakest of the 12 level 9 girls, not to mention the 6 level 10s and 7 elite gymnasts there. Alicia soon discovered that one thing her coaches had told her was indeed true. In the new gym, they were all business and expected tremendous effort out of every gymnast. For Alicia, this was like finally finding her way home after being lost. She was thrilled at the new gym's training regime and the coaches' demand for excellence. She immediately quit her old gym and committed herself to a two-hour commute every day just to train. She had found a perfect environment to pursue *her* goal.

Coaches and parents need to be aware of this important principle. The goal must belong to the athlete. Parents and coaches who push an athlete toward a goal that's more theirs than the athlete's are asking for trouble. This pushing is counterproductive and frequently causes performance difficulties and burnout for the athlete. Furthermore, even if the athlete does succeed, the success likely comes at a tremendous psychological and emotional cost. Multiple gold-medal diver Greg Louganis is a classic example. Pushed relentlessly by his father, Greg became one of the greatest divers in the history of the sport. Unfortunately, Louganis paid dearly for his success in the sport. Several years ago when he announced that he had the AIDS virus, he was also quoted as saying, "I wouldn't wish my life on anyone." This comment was directed at his father's overinvolvement, excessive pushing, and emotional abuse, all so Greg could become a champion.

As a coach, your job is to encourage your athletes to dream big and set challenging goals. You want to paint a picture for them of all that's possible and then help them reach *their* possibilities. You want to encourage them and sometimes even push them in this direction, so long as that's where *they* truly want to go. If you set *your* goals *for them*, and they refuse to buy into them, you'll end up frustrated, disappointed, and in constant conflict with your athletes.

You can still talk to your team about *your* tradition of winning and striving for personal excellence. You can put your goals and expectations clearly in front of your athletes, but you have to be sure that your team as a whole has a personal investment in these goals. One way to insure that your team as a whole identifies and then commits to common goals is by starting your season with a team goal party.

A goal party is simply a one- to two-hour team meeting dedicated to developing that season's goals. Everyone is encouraged to participate, and *all* the goals generated by discussion are written down, including the totally ridiculous ones, for example, "We should stay out late and party every night" or "Practice should be no more than 15 minutes." Next, ask your athletes to decide which of these goals they want to seriously commit to as a team, and then compile a second list. Have this list typed, copied, and passed out for each team member to sign. As the coach, you are now in a better position to know what your athletes want and can more effectively mold their goals in a direction that's congruent with your beliefs and coaching philosophy.

Principle #2—Break the Goal Into Manageable Parts

Goals, like a good map, can help you get where you want to go in the sport. They break down your journey into manageable parts. You take a huge, scary, and possibly overwhelming goal that may be in the distant future, your big-enough why, and chunk it down into intermediate- and short-term

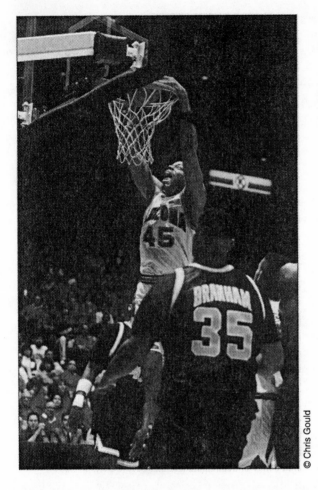

© Chris Gould

goals that you can work on daily, weekly, and monthly. When you approach any obstacle, slump, or big goal in this way, few goals or obstacles will be too big to handle.

Unfortunately, most athletes think goal setting is simply picking out the big, long-term goal. They decide one day, "I want to play pro ball," "I want to get a college scholarship," or "I want to set a high school record." Like that trip to San Francisco, their goal does not include any of the many smaller target destinations that accurately guide them "cross-country" to that ultimate goal. However, if you don't first figure out how exactly you're going to get out of Massachusetts and precisely where you'll go next, you may find yourself stuck in a swamp somewhere in the middle of the Florida Everglades as a gator's appetizer instead of where you wanted to go in California.

To make goal setting work for you, start by thinking of that ultimate destination. Where do you *really* want to go in the sport? Regardless of the slump you may be struggling with now, what do you want to achieve before you retire? The "Discovering That Superperformer Inside" exercise on page 194 will help you accomplish this first important task of identifying your overriding goal. Once you've thought of exactly what you'd like to accomplish, work backward to identify the skills and strengths you'll need to perform at this goal level. You can start by talking with or reading about athletes who have already achieved the goals that you desire. What do these athletes have mentally and physically that you don't yet possess? Assessing their physical and mental strengths will help you organize the intermediate goals necessary to reach your ultimate goal. You may need to develop greater physical strength and endurance. These successful athletes may have more advanced defensive and offensive skills in the sport than you presently have. As you think about the strengths of these athletes, you may realize that mental toughness is another area that you need to improve.

As you compare where you are right now with where you want to be, it's important to understand that each of your shortcomings will serve as a specific goal target for you to work on over the next few months and years. Be sure to check with a trusted coach who can help you fill in the blanks that may arise as you do this exercise. A good coach can help you map the journey so you get to your destination in the best way possible without wasting any more time or energy than necessary.

Once you have a good idea of what areas you need to develop, plan with your coach some long-term (one to three years or more), intermediate (six months to a year), and short-term (one to five months) goal targets. Then further break these short-term goals into weekly and daily goals. *The heart of winning goal setting is to connect what you are doing today in practice with where you ultimately want to go.*

Let's say, for example, that your goal is to get a full scholarship to play for a Division I basketball program. You just finished eighth grade, struggled with your confidence and shooting all last year, and have all of high school to work toward your dream. How can you snap out of your performance stagnation and break down your big-enough why into smaller pieces? Working backward, you realize that you won't have control over your physical height by the time you reach college age. That's an uncontrollable. However, you do have some control over the skill that you develop, your attitude, confidence, physical strength, and conditioning.

Connect what you are doing today in practice
with where you ultimately want to go.

Watching Division I players on TV or in person can give you a sense of what's needed to play at that level. Working with a knowledgeable coach can help you fill in the specific pieces of what you must accomplish over the next four years. Working backward from your long-term goal, you might identify manageable pieces something like the basketball player did in the following sample plan.

BREAKING DOWN A LONG-TERM GOAL

Note: Outcome goals are not italicized; process goals are.

■ Senior Year of High School

- Sign with one of three Division I schools seriously interested (all full-scholarship offers)
- First team, all-conference guard
- Starting guard on varsity team
- Set school records in assists and steals
- Lead team in assists, steals, and highest assists-to-turnovers ratio
- Reputation as defensive specialist and solid playmaker
- Average two 3-point shots made per game
- Average points per game: 15
- Free-throw percentage: 90%
- *4 hours of practice daily during the off-season (1 hour of free throws)*
- *10 minutes of mental rehearsal nightly (alternate mastery and coping imagery)*
- *5 to 10 minutes of relaxation training (any technique) nightly before games*
- *During daily free-throw practice, work on preshot ritual, staying in the now*

■ Summer Before Senior Year

- Qualify for blue-chip basketball camp
- *6 hours of practice daily (1-1/2 hours of free throws)*
- *Participate in summer league competition*
- *One-on-one work with Division I college player*
- *10 minutes of mental rehearsal nightly (alternate mastery and coping imagery)*
- *10 minutes of daily relaxation training (alternate breathing technique and progressive muscle relaxation)*
- *During daily free-throw practice, work on preshot ritual, staying in the now*

■ Junior Year of High School

- Starting guard on varsity team
- Team leader

- Lead team in assists and steals
- Average one 3-point shot made per game
- Average points per game: 10
- Free-throw percentage: 80%
- *3 hours of practice daily during the off-season (1 hour of free throws)*
- *10 minutes of mental rehearsal nightly (alternate mastery and coping imagery)*
- *10 minutes of relaxation training nightly before games*
- *5 minutes of daily concentration training*
- *During daily free-throw practice, work on preshot ritual, staying in the now*

■ Summer Before Junior Year

- *Attend three basketball camps*
- *5 hours of practice daily (1-1/4 hours of free throws)*
- *Participate in summer league competition*
- *One-on-one work with Division I player*
- *10 minutes of mental rehearsal nightly (alternate mastery and coping imagery)*
- *15 minutes of daily relaxation training*
- *5 minutes of daily concentration training (focus on breath and counting exercise)*
- *Perfect preshot ritual for free throws*
- *Develop and practice mistake ritual (several ministeps that help change focus, replace negative self-talk, and lower physiological arousal through quick relaxation techniques)*

■ Sophomore Year of High School

- Starting guard on junior varsity team
- Average seven assists and three steals per game
- Average 10 points per game
- Free-throw percentage: 75%
- *3 hours of daily practice during the off-season (45 minutes of free throws)*
- *15 minutes of mental rehearsal nightly (alternate mastery and coping imagery)*

→

- *15 minutes of relaxation training (progressive muscle relaxation)*
- *Practice focusing in the now of games and workouts*
- *Make and post positive affirmation cards*
- *Use positive self-talk daily to deal with mistakes and failures*

■ Summer Before Sophomore Year

- *Attend at least two basketball camps*
- *5 hours of daily practice (1 hour of free throws)*
- *Participate in summer league competition*
- *10 minutes of mental rehearsal daily (alternate mastery and coping imagery)*
- *15 minutes of relaxation training daily (progressive muscle relaxation)*
- *Practice focusing in the now during workouts (1 hour daily)*
- *Continue to work with victory log (a journal in which to record all the small victories or accomplishments achieved in a day, such as running extra sprints, mastering a new skill, being complimented by a coach, and so on)*
- *10 minutes of daily practice on positive reframing*

■ Freshman Year of High School

- Starting guard on junior varsity team
- Average three assists and two steals per game
- Average eight points per game
- Free-throw percentage: 70%
- *3 hours of daily off-season practice (45 minutes of free throws)*
- *Continue to set and use daily and weekly goal sheets*
- *10 minutes of nightly mental rehearsal practice (alternate mastery and coping imagery)*
- *Learn and practice 15 minutes daily one new relaxation technique*
- *Continue using victory log daily*
- *Watch for uncontrollables daily*

■ Summer Before Freshman Year

- *Attend at least two basketball camps*
- *4 hours of daily practice (1 hour of free throws)*

- *Participate in summer league competition*
- *Spend one full day developing detailed goal plan to bust slump and reach dream*
- *Develop a mastery script and make a mastery audiotape*
- *Mentally rehearse 10 minutes every other day using mastery tape*
- *Develop a coping script and make a coping audiotape*
- *Mentally rehearse 10 minutes every other day using coping tape*
- *Learn and practice one relaxation technique daily (15 minutes) to better handle nerves*
- *Start a victory log to turn around negative thinking*
- *Practice recognizing the uncontrollables (30 minutes per day)*

As a coach, teaching your athletes how to break their big-enough why into small, manageable parts is crucial to building confidence and fueling motivation. Having a clear objective and well-conceived plan of how to accomplish that objective, whether the goal is to overcome a long-term slump or make the starting varsity, fortifies the athlete with a sense of purpose. Furthermore, with each successful step taken toward that objective, the athlete's confidence grows. Help your athletes focus their efforts on accomplishing these small, manageable pieces. If they're struggling, help them attack the slump both physically and mentally every day, one small piece at time. (Refer to the sample goal plan above.)

Principle #3—Set Deadlines for Your Goals

There's nothing like a good deadline to get the adrenaline flowing and yourself mobilized. Attaching a timeline to your short-, intermediate-, and long-term goals will add a sense of urgency that is critical for the goal-setting process to work for you. Without a deadline, you'll have difficulty disciplining yourself. A goal of "making the varsity" does not carry the same degree of urgency as "making the varsity by *next season*." If you know *when* the goal has to be accomplished, you will be more likely to give up that summer at the beach to train daily. A deadline helps you prioritize your efforts and keeps your focus on the important task at hand. That way, when your friends call and encourage you to blow off training for the week, knowing how much time you have left helps you consistently make a decision that fits your true priorities.

A deadline helps you prioritize your efforts and keeps your focus on the important task at hand.

The deadlines that you attach to your goals make them more compelling and real. It's easier to take action and channel your energies when you can feel the immediacy of an approaching target date. In these time-pressured situations, you won't simply try to accomplish your goal—you'll do *whatever is necessary* to accomplish it.

A word of caution here. Setting a deadline to get through a slump, an outcome goal (Principle # 4), could be counterproductive and may actually keep you stuck longer. The sense of urgency produced by the deadline can generate more pressure on you than is useful. Set time goals for accomplishing each step in your plan or for mastering the slump-busting skills (process goals). Having a timeline is useful. However, if you focus your energies on accomplishing these process goals, you will bust the slump as a result.

Creating training deadlines and fostering a sense of urgency is an important coaching tool that helps athletes stay on track and put more into their training. Coaches will frequently push their athletes to go beyond their perceived limits by setting goal deadlines. When used appropriately, your deadlines can become a critically important motivational tool leading to peak performance. As an example, a coach tells her team after their goal-setting party, "If we want to win the championship, we have to be in this kind of shape (coach details this) and have acquired these specific skills (coach details these) by this particular date (coach specified date). Ladies, that means we have only four months to get ourselves there. Let's get cracking!"

However, as a coach, avoid using deadlines with your players who are struggling with a performance slump. For example, coaches who pressure their skaters, divers, or gymnasts to get over a fear-based block by a specific deadline inadvertently cause their athletes more performance problems. The athletes become even more impatient with themselves and distracted by the coach's pressure, deepening their troubles.

Principle #4—Use Both Outcome and Process Goals

Some of the goals in the previous basketball player's timeline are outcome oriented, for example, scoring 15 points per game, averaging so many assists or steals, making a team, and so on. Others are *process* oriented (in *italics* in the sample plan), such as spending a certain amount of time each day practicing, developing and using a victory log, training with a more skilled player, and so on. You'll notice that in the beginning, this athlete set more process than outcome goals. For example, in his freshman and sophomore years, he had six process and four outcome goals. This shifted slightly in his junior year (five process and six outcome) and then more dramatically in his senior year (four process and nine outcome). During the summers, all his goals were process-focused until his senior year.

Process goals are your key to athletic success and slump busting. They involve things that you can directly control, like skill development (like learning to dribble with both hands, to throw a curve, or to stay relaxed under pressure), time invested in practicing (for example, running for one hour daily, shooting three-pointers for 30 minutes, or doing 10 minutes of mental rehearsal daily), number of repetitions per skill (such as shooting 500 free throws each day or hitting 200 crosscourt backhands twice a day), and all the short-term things you need to do to increase your chances of accomplishing the outcome goals.

> ***P****rocess goals are your key to athletic success
> and slump busting.*

Outcome goals are frequently out of your direct control as an athlete. You have no direct control over whether you'll make the team, start, score a certain number of goals, or win the championship. *Remember, overemphasis on outcome goals can cause a slump.* You must learn to think less about *what* you want to accomplish and more about *how* you'll accomplish it. Thinking about

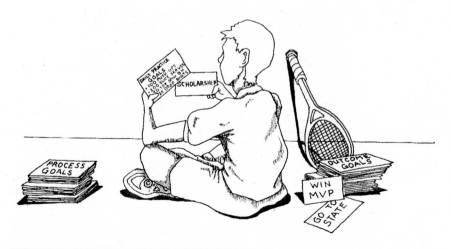

Use outcome and process goals.

your outcome goals *while* you're performing will pressure you into performing poorly and distract your concentration from a peak-performance focus.

Occasionally, all an athlete needs to successfully bust a slump is to change goal focus during competition from outcome to process. For example, Mike was a professional golfer struggling with his game. He'd play well until a mistake or two cost him some strokes. Then he'd become overly concerned with his score and the strokes he'd have to make up, while he was preparing for his next shot. For example, over an eight-foot putt, he'd think, "I'm down three strokes. I've gotta make this to save par." This goal focus caused him to tighten up and blow the shot. But Mike was in good company. In 1989, golf pro Scott Hoch did the same thing over a two-foot putt that would have won him the Master's title. Hoch's final thoughts before this putt were goal directed: "This is for all the marbles."

Mike was able to get his game back on track and snap his slump when he switched his outcome goals on the course to process goals. Instead of keeping score on each shot, he worked on his concentration over the ball. Focusing on the ball and certain swing cues are process-related goals and totally in the golfer's control. So Mike started "scoring" his concentration over the

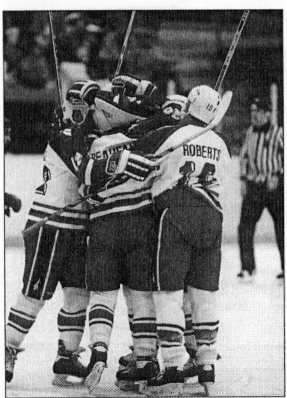

© Claus Andersen

ball. Before each shot, his process goal was to *feel* his swing cue while he watched the ball. He began to rate his concentration on a scale of 1 to 10 for each shot. If he could feel his back foot planted properly as he was swinging, then he would give himself a 10. If he was thinking about the shot's outcome or his score while he was hitting, he'd give himself a 2 or 3. The higher Mike scored in concentration (a process goal), the better he played and the lower he actually scored (outcome goal). Like Mike, to increase the likelihood of reaching your outcome goal and snapping a slump, you must refocus your energy and attention on achieving *process* goals.

As a coach, encourage your athletes to set outcome goals and then help them develop and use process goals daily as a vehicle to reach their dreams. Building upper-body strength or confidence are outcomes that you can orchestrate by focusing your athletes on the daily and weekly repetition of specific exercises and techniques that will help them acquire these outcomes. For example, 200 push-ups a day, weight machines three times a week for one hour, daily use of a victory log, and 10 minutes daily of positive reframing are all specific process goals that can help athletes achieve their outcome goals.

You can use outcome goals to remind your athletes why they are out there, their big-enough why. Such a reminder will motivate them to maintain a high level of intensity in the face of the physical and mental hardships of intense training. Use process goals with them in practice to help them develop mental and physical skills.

During competition, your major task as a coach is to keep your athletes focused entirely on process goals (see Step 3). You do that by assigning each athlete specific jobs to do (for example, rebound quickly from mistakes, box out under the boards, keep your hands loose on the bat, or make the extra pass as a team). By keeping your athletes away from an outcome focus, you'll paradoxically increase the chances that they'll achieve the desired outcome.

Principle #5—Make Your Goals Specific

Many athletes fail at goal setting because they don't make their goals specific. Wanting to get better, faster, stronger, or more talented are goals that are too general to be helpful. Goals are supposed to guide your efforts. If the direction or destination is unclear, the result will be unclear. Goals are like the homing device on a guided missile. They program your energy in a particular direction until you hit the target. However, if the homing device is set on an indistinct target, the missile, being unguided, will fly all over the place until the engine burns out.

Even a goal of playing professional baseball is too vague to really be useful. You could play a minor role on a minor league team as a professional and never see the inside of a major league ballpark. You could make a major league team and sit on the bench, or you could be a productive member of the starting lineup. Which do you *really* want? The more specific you can be about your goals, the more likely you are to reach them. The high school basketball player we discussed with the dream of playing Division I basketball clearly demonstrated this important goal-setting principle. Not only was his goal of getting a full scholarship quite specific, but so too were all his important intermediate goals.

Coaches need to help athletes set specific, detailed goals. If an athlete or team presents you with goals that are too vague, press them for more detail until they know exactly what they want. Especially for setting process goals *during* competition, the more specific you can get your athletes to be on their game goals, the more likely they'll have a successful performance. This concept coincides with a basic principle of effective coaching: The clearer and more detailed your instructions to your athletes, the easier it is for them to accomplish the desired task.

Principle #6—Keep Your Goals Flexible

When missing, unclear, or used incorrectly, your goals can get you totally lost. They can lead you toward a slump and frustrate you into giving up on your dream and quitting the sport. To keep yourself going in the right direction, use your goals as a map, nothing more. In other words, be flexible with your use of them. If you fail to make a goal, then adjust that goal and immediately set another one. If you reach a goal quicker than you expected, then set another, more challenging one.

For example, if your big goal is to play college basketball, but as a 12-year-old, you get cut from the traveling team, you must learn to handle this temporary setback constructively. Don't view it as a failure and excuse for leaving the sport. Perhaps you need to improve your dribbling and ball-handling skills. Maybe you need to work harder on your shooting. Maybe the goal of making the team was unrealistic at this time. Failure to reach *any* goal along the way should be used as feedback for how to get closer to that ultimate goal. Just because you take a wrong turn or two, you don't have to cancel the whole trip and go home. Where would the basketball world and sneaker sales be if Michael Jordan, who was cut from his high school team, had given up because of his failure to reach his goal of playing varsity ball?

Remember, as you work toward putting your performance difficulties behind you, use your goals as a flexible tool to guide you rather than as a fence to lock you in. If something goes wrong along the way, blame the goals, not yourself. As you go through the goal-setting process to bust out of that slump, try more than just one or two steps in the model.

Chrissey was a swimmer who had been in the performance doldrums for almost two years, consistently swimming below her potential. Her expectations and goals were continually getting in her way. She was a perfectionist, a driven athlete who always demanded the best from herself. By itself, perfectionism isn't necessarily bad. You can't reach your potential as an athlete unless you're willing to stretch yourself and continually strive for the next level. If you're satisfied with mediocrity, you'll go nowhere. This drive to be the best can be found in *every* successful athlete. This wasn't Chrissey's problem. Her troubles stemmed from not completely understanding the function that her goals were supposed to play in her development as an athlete.

To Chrissey, goals were etched in stone. You set and then reached them, or you were a failure. Because of this thinking, she put too much pressure on herself whenever she competed. If she won a race but didn't swim as fast as she expected, Chrissey would get down on herself and see this win as a loss. She was constantly measuring her performances with her goals and outcome expectations. However, instead of using this checking-back process as a way to keep herself on track and moving toward her dreams, Chrissey would do it in a negative, self-critical, and pressured way.

In practice she would obsess about her goals: "Am I going fast enough?" "Will I make the cuts?" "I should be going faster than Jenny!" "Why am I slower than last year?" At competitions she'd continue this narrow focus on her goals, a focus that proved to be extremely performance-disrupting. Chrissey hadn't yet learned that she should never take her outcome-based goals into a performance. These goals need to be left safely in the locker room. While they may be critical for motivation *in practice*, the goals' outcome focus put Chrissey too much in her head when she competed and distracted her from the important tasks at hand.

During her slump, before she physically raced, Chrissey's mind did some racing of its own across all the possibilities of not reaching her goals: "What if I don't get this time set?" "What if she beats me?" "What if I don't qualify today? I'll only have two more chances." "I gotta do this under 11 minutes or else!" This overemphasis on her outcome goals distracted her concentration and tied her in mental and physical knots. As a result, she swam mechanically and poorly. Her slow times further frustrated and angered her. She knew she *should* be swimming faster and felt like a failure that she wasn't moving closer to her goals the way she thought she *should.* These frustrations only

→

caused her to further increase her self-imposed pressure, getting her more stuck.

Chrissey was finally able to interrupt this negative cycle and break her slump by using goals more effectively. First, I taught her that to reach her outcome goals, she must focus all her energies on her process goals. Since she didn't have any specific process goals, we started with formulating some. Through our discussions, she realized that her concentration, self-talk, and prerace nerves were part of the problem. As a result, she developed process goals to work on these three areas in practice and at home. For concentration, she set a goal to swim mentally in the now every other set in practice. At home, she set a goal to practice controlling her focus 5 minutes daily. For her negative self-talk, she set goals to use thought-stopping and reframing 10 minutes a day both in and outside of practice. In addition, she set a goal to practice a relaxation exercise before bed every night for three weeks.

For her races, we changed her goal focus so that, instead of worrying about the outcome, she concentrated on the process goals of feeling her pace and keeping her stroke turnover fast and smooth. With those two new goals in mind and with the help of the other skills she had acquired, Chrissey broke through her slump. Two months after first rearranging her goals, Chrissey had five lifetime best swims in a qualifying meet for the Massachusetts Bay State Games.

Let's say, for example, that fears are fueling your performance problems. You pick up this book and anxiously turn right to Step 4 on handling fears. You set an outcome goal for yourself to eliminate your fears in four weeks, and then you take the six fear-busting strategies and set process goals to exclusively practice each strategy for four days. After the four weeks, your fears, although somewhat smaller, are still incapacitating. Are you a failure? Is the slump-busting model ineffectual? No! You simply need to re-examine your goals. Perhaps the outcome goal of solving your problem in so short a time was unrealistic. Maybe your impatience to be rid of the slump caused you to set process goals that were too limiting. Perhaps you need to work with additional slump-busting strategies by starting with the process goal of reading the entire book. When you don't get what you want, examine and then reset your goals.

As a coach, this principle is important in helping your athletes constructively manage and use their failures. Failure to reach a goal should not be used as a reflection of the athlete's or team's ability or worth. Instead, failures should be used as learning experiences, as a time to go back to the

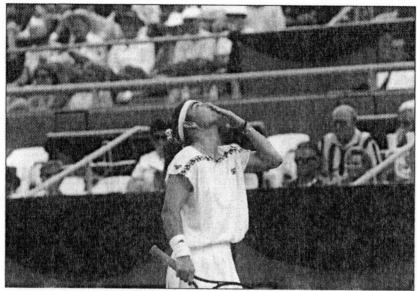

© Robert Skeoch

drawing board to figure out what worked and what didn't. When framed in this way, failure should stimulate new goals and renewed determination and motivation. Help your athletes understand this concept of goals as flexible guides, not as rigid markers of success and failure.

Principle #7—Frame Your Goals in a Positive Way

If I said to you, "Close your eyes right now, and whatever you do, don't think about pink elephants," you'd probably notice a pastel pachyderm dancing around in your head. Similarly, when a coach yells to an athlete, "Don't foul!" the athlete inadvertently finds his mind playing with images of fouling. So when the keeper goes into the game and sets as her goal "I'm not going to let anyone beat me today," her focus is being drawn in the wrong direction.

When you frame your goals negatively in this manner, you may end up getting exactly what you don't want. A negative frame, as we discussed in Step 6, conjures up the wrong pictures and doesn't spell out what you *do* want. Since the images that you create in your mind's eye preprogram your performance, it is critical that your goals lead you to see what you want to happen. Goals like "I don't want to be nervous in big games" or "I don't want to be intimidated when I play this opponent" not only call up the negative, but they also set an unclear target. Instead, when you set your goals, spell out specifically what you *want* rather than *don't want* to happen. For example, the soccer goalie should set for herself process goals like being in the right position and maintaining her intensity and focus throughout the game.

If slumping athletes set negative goals, their goals will only maintain their performance difficulties. Slumping athletes may be unaware that they have set a negative target for themselves. Goals like "I don't want to drop the ball again," "I won't strike out with the bases loaded," and "I don't want to die in the last 100 meters" subconsciously focus the athlete negatively. After golfer Greg Norman's painful collapse on the final day of the 1996 Masters after dominating the field, and his history of last-day fades in the big ones, he must have had to work hard to keep the negative goal of "not blowing my lead again" from sneaking into his consciousness the last day of his next important tournament. To more effectively bust that slump, set goals that steer you *away* from your problem and *toward* the solution. Use the exercise below to practice positively reframing negative goals.

> **S**et goals that steer you away from your problem and toward the solution.

Your job as a coach is to teach your athletes to focus on and go after what they want. Be quick to interrupt their natural tendency to gravitate toward the negative. Use the following exercise or develop your own more sports-specific exercise to give your players practice in turning negative goals positive.

MAKING YOUR GOALS POSITIVE

Take the following negative goals and reframe them positively. Possible answers appear at the end of the exercise.

Negative Goal	Positive Reframe
Example:	
I don't want to get cut.	I will make the team.

1. We won't lose again in the quarterfinals.
2. I don't want to blow my lead.
3. We won't get intimidated.
4. I won't get too nervous.
5. We won't let their offense run all over us.
6. I won't let myself get distracted by crowd noise.
7. I don't want to get stuck on the bench.
8. I won't let the refs' calls get to me.

9. I don't want to hang onto my mistakes.
10. We won't make any stupid mistakes.

Possible answers:
  1. We will win it all this year.
  2. I will finish the competition strong.
  3. We will play confidently.
  4. I will stay calm and composed.
  5. We will shut their offense down.
  6. I will stay focused on my stick handling.
  7. I will be a starter by the third game.
  8. I will let bad calls go immediately.
  9. I will quickly rebound from my mistakes.
  10. We will play a smart game.

Principle #8—Make Your Goals Measurable

One purpose of setting goals is to motivate you through successive achievement of one small goal after another. Each accomplishment increases your confidence and motivates you to move on to the next destination in the journey. For this process to work, these accomplishments must be measurable. You have to *know* that you're moving in the right direction. Easily measurable markers along the path provide feedback about your progress.

Measurable goals go hand in hand with specific goals. Being able to do 100 push-ups, bench press your own weight, and run the 100-yard dash in 10.5 seconds are easily measurable goals. Similarly, sinking 15 out of 20 free-throw attempts, kicking 20 field goals in a row from 35 yards out, and clearing six feet on the high jump are more useful goals than shooting better, kicking more consistently, and jumping higher.

Having measurable goals is especially important as you work on busting your slump. While you may not be able to see immediate performance changes, you can measure, for example, the 10 minutes of daily practice of coping imagery, the 60 repetitions daily of your positive affirmation, the 12 times today that you moved toward instead of away from your fears, and the 20 minutes you spent in practice keeping yourself focused on the "now." Achieving these small, measurable slump-busting goals will increase your confidence and optimism about reaching the ultimate goal of beating the slump.

T he continual achievement of small successes fuels motivation and enhances self-confidence.

Coaches can be instrumental in building self-confidence by using this goal-setting principle. If you help your athletes construct their goals so that they are both specific and measurable, then the athletes can more easily see their progress. This continual achievement of small successes fuels motivation and enhances self-confidence. Clearly measurable goals allow this process to happen. Furthermore, by making your athletes set measurable goals, you can more easily short-circuit the negative cycle that snags perfectionist athletes when they ignore their successes. When perfectionist athletes reach a specific, measurable goal, they will have a hard time denying their success since it is right in front of them.

Principle #9—Write Your Goals Down and Post Them

When you aim your attention and energy toward a particular goal, your focus will help you mobilize your resources to turn this fantasy (all goals

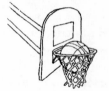

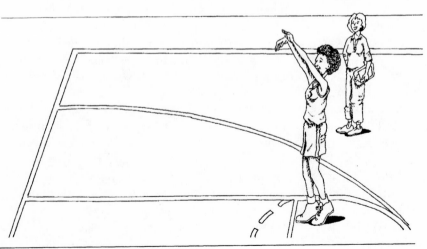

Make goals measurable.

start off as fantasy) into reality. Your continual thoughts about this goal, however far out it may be, add color, shape, and detail to the vague outline of this dream.

Writing your goals down takes this process one step further. The adage "Don't just think them, ink them" adds another important dimension to developing goals that really work for you. By writing your goals down and posting them in plain view, you formalize the contract you've made with yourself. This written commitment holds more motivational power for you than one that you simply whisper in the back of your mind. Furthermore, frequently seeing this commitment reminds you daily of the path you've chosen. It helps you order your priorities, focus your efforts, and direct your action.

In addition to posting your goals in an easily visible place, be sure to check off those short- and intermediate-term goals as you accomplish them. These accomplishments, no matter how small, provide you daily concrete evidence of your progress and growing success. This feedback is especially important if you're slumping and are hard-pressed to find anything positive in your performance.

Coaches who put up slogans around the locker room like "If you fail to plan, you're planning to fail," "Total effort from all members," and "Winners honor their commitments to themselves and their teammates" are indirectly using this goal-setting principle by reminding their athletes of important process goals: plan ahead, play as a team, and be committed. If the coach regularly preaches these goals, then the signs will have an even more positive impact on the team. Similarly, coaches can post specific team goals in clearly visible places around the training environment to keep their athletes focused on the team's big-enough why.

Sample Goals

By following these nine principles of effective goal setting, coaches and athletes will increase motivation, build confidence, and systematically create success. For the slumping athlete or team, these principles can help organize the slump-busting efforts so that they will pay off. Two examples follow. In the first, I will highlight some sample outcome and process goals for a slumping athlete, a softball player who has gone hitless for two months. She suffers from low self-confidence, negative thinking, and expectations of failure. In addition, her anxiety when she hits is performance-disrupting. (See Step 10.) In the second example, I will present some sample process and outcome goals for a team.

SAMPLE SLUMP-BUSTING INDIVIDUAL GOALS

■ Outcome Goals

- Become a highly confident hitter by season's end (5 months).
- Be calm and composed at the plate and in the field under pressure.
- Get batting average over .320 by end of season.
- Develop a positive attitude about my game, hitting, fielding, and place on the team (5 months).
- Rebound quickly from bad at-bats and bad games.

■ Process Goals

- Finish reading *Sports Slump Busting* by [date].
- Make a list of all my uncontrollables by 6:00 P.M. tonight.
- Keep a journal of negative self-talk starting today for seven straight days.
- Start a victory log and spend five minutes nightly making entries.
- Develop five affirmations, post them around my room, and put copies in equipment bag, on bat, and in glove.
- Work on reframing negative self-talk daily for two weeks in practice.
- Practice focus exercise three minutes nightly for one week (no distractions).
- Practice focus exercise with distractions three minutes nightly for two weeks.
- Practice relaxation exercise 10 minutes at bedtime first two weeks.
- Practice progressive muscle relaxation 15 minutes at bedtime second two weeks.
- Write a mastery script by next Tuesday.
- Record mastery script with music by following Sunday.
- Practice mastery imagery (three weeks from now) 10 minutes nightly for three weeks, emphasizing confidence and positive attitude.
- Practice mastery imagery using tape 10 minutes nightly for three weeks, emphasizing composure under pressure and relaxation at the plate.
- Make a coping script by Wednesday.
- Record coping script by Saturday.

- Practice coping imagery using tape 10 minutes on nongame nights, emphasizing composure under pressure and quick rebounding from mistakes.
- Develop mistake ritual and use in practice at least four times a day.
- Practice playing in the now in workouts 10 minutes daily.

SAMPLE SLUMP-BUSTING TEAM GOALS

■ Outcome Goals

- Win conference championship.
- Finish in top eight in state tourney (make quarterfinal round).
- Place five players on all-conference team.
- Beat the Cougars.
- Maintain 3.0 GPA team average.
- Get along well as a team all season.
- Achieve 90% or better participation in off-season weight training.
- All members maintain a positive attitude at practice and games.
- Achieve 100% individual offensive and defensive skill improvement across team.
- Achieve 100% commitment to team goals.

■ Process Goals

- All members participate once weekly in 30 minute team-building rap session.
- All members attend two nonsport outings or retreats this year.
- All members participate in mental toughness training sessions three times per week (imagery and relaxation).
- All members meet for team meals three times weekly.
- Members always take personal problems directly to teammate involved.
- All members focus on controllables daily.
- Teammates treat each other with respect every day.
- All members stay in the here and now in practice and games.
- Everyone smiles daily.

Working Toward Your Big-Enough Why

Let's apply the principles of winning goal setting to your slump-busting efforts. Athletes mired in slumps usually become conditioned to focus on their troubles and how stuck they feel. Such a problem focus only tends to kill motivation and increase despair. By deliberately switching your focus of attention away from the problem and toward the solution, you can get back in touch with the powerful inner resources that are always at your disposal. It's these resources that can ultimately help you break the slump and return to optimal performance.

To begin this solution-focused switch, think about your ultimate goal or big-enough why. What's your dream? This is the vehicle that will help transport you from the pits to the peak. Your big-enough why will provide you with the staying power to prevail when your road gets rocky and cluttered with obstacles. The following exercise is designed to emotionally move you away from your slump and get you more in touch with your inner strengths and resources. The exercise will heighten the emotional pull of your why. It will make your goals more real. The more emotion you attach to your why, the stronger its influence in helping you turn your dreams into reality.

DISCOVERING THAT SUPERPERFORMER INSIDE

Find a place free from distractions where you'll be undisturbed for 15 to 20 minutes. If you're an athlete working alone, make an audiotape of the following exercise so that you can do it carefully and slowly with your eyes closed. If you're a coach, then simply take your athletes through the exercise. A series of dots (. . .) means a 2 to 3 second pause.

Sitting or lying down comfortably, close your eyes and allow a few minutes to consider each of these preliminary questions:

1. What is your ultimate dream, your big-enough why? State in *positive terms* what you *want*, not what you *don't want*. Be as *specific* as possible. How far in the future does your goal lie? What year do you want to reach it? Consider in detail how you'll perform, act, talk, and feel if you achieve that big-enough why. Take your time to see, hear, and feel every part of your answer.

2. Now briefly consider where you are today. If you're stuck in a slump, are you gaining anything from staying stuck? (No one would deliberately choose to go into a slump. However, sometimes there are benefits that can come from getting stuck. For example, being in a slump can lower people's expectations of you and relieve some of the pressure.) Be honest with yourself here.

3. Can you remember performing at your peak? Briefly think back to this experience in as much detail as possible. How would you compare this peak performance to how you'll be able to perform once you reach your big-enough why?

4. Once you've achieved your big-enough why, how will your life be different? What effect will this achievement have on you and the people in your life? Where will you live? How will you feel about yourself? Will *Sports Illustrated* be calling for a cover shot? What will your days look like? How will you spend your time?

■ Exercise

1. Relax

Allow your mind to slowly empty and shift your focus of attention to your breathing. . . . Follow your breath in and out and feel yourself slow down inside. . . . You don't have to change your breathing at all. . . . Just inhale and exhale effortlessly as you sit or lie comfortably, focusing on your breathing. . . .

While you do this, mentally take yourself to a favorite place in your mind's eye. . . . Whether you "travel" to a beach, a cabin in the mountains, a lake, or the comfort of your own room doesn't matter. All that matters is that you find a relaxing place. . . . This place can be imaginary. . . or real. It can be up in the clouds or down to earth. . . . What's important about this place is that you feel safe there. . . . Look around. . . . What can you see? . . . familiar movements? . . . specific colors? . . . Do you associate certain sounds with this place? . . . sensations and feelings? . . . like a breeze, the warmth of the sun, the softness of grass, or a bed under you? . . .

2. Meet Your Superperformer Inside (SPI), That Future You Who Has Achieved Your Big-Enough Why

As you remain in that comfortable place, imagine that you can see your Superperformer Inside (SPI). Your SPI represents the you that

→

you're growing to become . . . your future or ideal you . . . the athlete who represents the achievement of your big dream. Watching this athlete from a comfortable distance, carefully study everything about him [her]. . . . His [her] appearance. . . build . . . walk . . . voice . . . and movements. . . . What can you learn about this future you that you're growing into? . . . Give your imagination free reign as you let the details of this person develop. . . . This athlete represents your inner potential . . . that superathlete who is developing inside you right now. . . . Spend some time examining your SPI's face. . . .

3. Look at Your Present Self

Imagine that you can look at your Present Self (PS) as if watching yourself in a mirror. . . . In as much detail as possible and without any judgments, look at your face, body, posture, and dress. . . . Study these images . . . your voice tone, volume, and tempo . . . your movements and mannerisms. . . . Notice how you interact with those around you . . . how you move. . . .

4. Compare Your Present Self (PS) With Your Superperformer Inside (SPI)

Look back to that future self (SPI) and notice the differences between him [her] and your present self. As you again carefully study this very competent athlete, what can you learn? . . . Watch this SPI perform. . . . Watch the smoothness and power of the movements . . . the skill execution . . . the strength and speed. . . . Notice how your SPI's performance differs from your present performance. Have your SPI flawlessly repeat a specific movement over and over to get a real sense of these differences. Perhaps one thing that stands out as you study your SPI is the confidence and relaxation in his [her] movements.

5. Become Your SPI

Imagine that your SPI can walk over to you and introduce himself [herself] . . . perhaps even explain to you that he [she] is here from the future and is the you that you're growing to become. As he [she] reaches up and shakes your hand, imagine you can flow completely into his [her] image . . . so that you can actually *become* your SPI. . . . You begin to feel what he [she] feels . . . hear through his [her] ears . . . see the world through his [her] eyes. . . . You join him [her] so completely that you even have access to all his [her] memories. . . . What obstacles and setbacks did you overcome? . . . What disappointments have you bounced back from? . . . Experience what this is like in as much detail as possible. How do you now carry yourself? . . . speak? . . . What does your confidence level feel like? . . . In detail, experience how it feels to perform with your new capabilities . . . the smoothness . . . the ease . . . the power . . . the effortlessness of your movements. . . . As this SPI right now, what do you believe about yourself and your abilities? . . . How does it feel to have this level of mental toughness? . . . Experience fully what it's like to have achieved your big-enough why. . . .

6. Develop an SPI Cue

As you experience fully being your future self right now, come up with a *cue* or reminder of this SPI state. Your reminder can be the feeling you get when you hold your head high, the way your SPI does . . . or breathe deeper. . . . It can be a particular image that you see, like a close-up of your face as this SPI. . . . It can be a word or phrase that you repeat to yourself that captures the SPI experience. . . . It can be a physical movement that you make, like a fist. Whatever you choose for that reminder, feel deeply what it's like to have achieved that big-enough why, and as you do, repeat your cue to yourself. Repeat the sequence of experiencing deeply the feeling of being this SPI. Then use your cue several times to bring back the experience. . . .

Let go of your images briefly . . . and as you do . . . understand that your experience of this SPI or future self is *very real*. To see, hear, and feel it in your imagination, the neural patterns in your brain must already exist as part of your behavior right now. In other words, important parts of this future self already exist inside of you. . . . They are therefore available to you as a powerful resource to help you turn your big-enough why into reality.

7. Recapture Your SPI

As you sit or lie comfortably, use your cue to again recapture the sights, sounds, and feelings of this future self. Do this in detail, as if you could turn the dials of experience up so that everything is bright, clear, loud, and vivid. . . . Sit with your SPI for a few more seconds and then once more let the image fade. . . . Take a deep breath, and as you exhale . . . let yourself relax even more. . . . Then one last time use your cue to bring back the future you, so that you experience fully your SPI. . . . Study the images and feelings . . . everything about this experience . . . how powerful you can make it now . . . and then effortlessly memorize all these feelings, thoughts, images, and sensations for future use, as you practice becoming that superperformer inside.

Take a few minutes to reorient yourself. Then make a list of the resources, strengths, and skills that you were able to experience from your "meeting" with your SPI. When you examined yourself after having reached your big-enough why, how were you different? What did you discover about your SPI? How can you use goal setting to help you acquire these internal resources and skills so they become directly available to you? For example, if you were impressed with your future self's mental toughness or physical stamina, how can you work on these skills as minigoals in your daily training? The more detailed you can make these images of this future self, the clearer your path to your goals will become and the more motivated you'll be to start your journey along that path.

Conclusion

"Divide and conquer" is an effective military strategy. As you square off against that slump, you can use this strategy to win this battle. Through the systematic and correct use of goal setting, you can move your athletic performance from the outhouse to the penthouse. Guided by the principles of peak performance, you can eliminate, one at a time, the mental mistakes and weaknesses that keep the slump intact. In their place, you can substitute mental toughness. Furthermore, you can use your newly acquired skills in goal setting to get back on track toward your ultimate athletic dream.

In the next step of the slump-busting model, we will continue to strengthen your positive belief in yourself that you developed in Step 5. Step 8 will teach you how to take your self-confidence to a winning level. Successful athletes are supremely confident in themselves, no matter what. Setbacks and failures do not shake this confidence. What will happen to your performance when you harness your confidence? Let's find out.

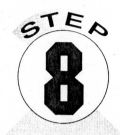

BUILDING
SELF-CONFIDENCE

*"The fight is won or lost far away from witnesses . . .
behind the lines, in the gym, and out there on the
road, long before I dance under those lights."*

—Muhammad Ali

As your slump begins to lose its grip on you, you'll find your attitude begins to change. The previous steps in the model will have helped you turn your negative thinking and low self-confidence around so that you start to believe in yourself again. Regaining control (Step 2) and learning how to develop a championship focus (Step 3) will have helped you put the skids to the slump by increasing your confidence and reducing your preperformance stress. Directly challenging and neutralizing slump-fueling fears (Step 4) and learning to expect success (Step 5) will add to a growing sense of control. You're back on track and building up positive momentum.

Your self-confidence and movement away from a slump mentality is further enhanced through consistent use of positive imagery (Step 6). As you begin to more regularly see what you want to happen, a success cycle replaces the slump-based failure cycle. The effective use of goal setting (Step 7) further drives this performance-enhancing cycle.

As you enter this next step in the model, you will learn how to build on the confidence you've already established. Strengthening your self-confidence will provide a solid base for mental toughness, an opposite mind-set to a slump mentality.

Confidence-feeding mental toughness is present in all great athletes. They have an inner sense that no matter what happens, they are up to the task. This kind of confidence is blind to failures and setbacks. It pays no heed to physical limitations or handicaps. It ignores the negativity and testimony of "experts" who say failure awaits the athlete's futile efforts. While confidence may temporarily wane within great athletes, it can't be extinguished. Sooner or later it's burning brighter than ever, illuminating the path to eventual success.

The confidence of a champion is visible and infectious. Teammates and opponents alike can feel it. Teammates of football great Joe Montana *knew* that when he started another last-minute, back-to-the-wall drive, they were going to win. Montana's confidence affected everyone on the field. It made the 49ers better and intimidated their opponents. It created an illusion of inevitability that wore the opposition down. The same thing happens when the Chicago Bulls' Michael Jordan is on the floor. If the game is on the line and the Bulls are faltering, opposing teams *know* that he's going to take over the game in the remaining minutes and rob them of the win. Jordan is unstoppable, and his confidence screams out loud and clear that he will find a way to lead his team to victory. Where can you get this kind of self-confidence?

Some athletes erroneously think that confidence like this comes solely from previous success. You play a great match, finally make the team, run a fantastic race at state, or have the game of your life, and now you have some basis for feeling confident. It is true that successful experiences are tremendous confidence boosters. Nothing can make you feel quite as good about yourself as that big win or achieving a huge goal. However, does this mean that you can't feel true confidence without first having an experience of success? Absolutely not! Olympic swimmer Tom Dolan wasn't USA #1 when he started signing his name that way. Muhammad Ali certainly wasn't the greatest when he first began to tell everyone that he was. In the beginning, having an inner trust in yourself and your athletic potential does not require proof.

> **Y**ou can grow strength and confidence out of physical hardship, frustration, deprivation, and failure.

There's a saying used in most endurance sports: "Anything that doesn't kill you will make you stronger." Unpleasant experiences in training and in life can indeed provide you with the opportunity to get smarter and tougher. You can grow strength and confidence out of physical hardship, frustration, deprivation, and failure. All you need to do is to recognize these uncomfortable situations for the *confidence-developing opportunities* that they are, and then seize them.

When 1996 Olympic swimmer Tom Dolan was a kid, he would regularly sign his name "Tom Dolan, USA #1." This wasn't simply an act of empty bravado. Young Dolan was convinced that what he was signing would someday come true. He was that confident. Some might have thought that the boy was a deluded dreamer. Having a big goal is not a bad thing for a youngster. However, this dream seemed impractical in this case. Young Dolan had a serious case of exercise-induced asthma and a constricted breathing passage. These physical liabilities limited his oxygen intake to a mere 20 percent of normal. In a grueling, endurance-based sport like swimming, only having one-fifth the lung capacity of your competitors puts you at a serious disadvantage. As a baseball player, golfer, or even a high jumper, he may have gotten away with these limitations. But as a swimmer? Not a chance! Perhaps his difficulty getting oxygen affected his brain!

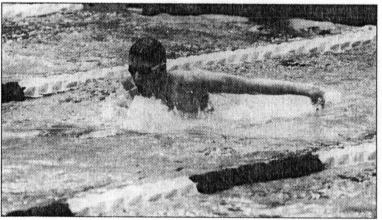

© University of Michigan/Bob Kalmbach

When Tom Dolan was 15, he won three titles at the junior nationals. When he was 18 and the youngest male member of the U.S. team, he set the world record in the 400 IM while winning the event at the world championships in Rome. In his three seasons at the University of Michigan, he set three U.S. records and was twice named NCAA swimmer of the year. At the 1996 Olympic Trials, Dolan put his swimming where his signature was. In the 400 IM, the sport's most grueling race, he swam the fastest time ever in the U.S. and the third-fastest time in history! At the Atlanta Olympics, he beat college teammate Eric Namesnik to win a gold medal in this event. *Tom Dolan, USA #1.*

Physical Preparation

A coach once told me, "If you want something badly enough and you're willing to work for it, you'll eventually get it." Is this the secret to growing championship self-confidence? If you *want* something badly enough and you're *willing to work for it*, is the sky really the limit? Does this explain major league pitcher Jim Abbott's success, despite the physical limitation of having only one hand? Is that why Boston Celtic legend Larry Bird's critics used to say, "Sure, he's a great ballplayer, but he only has average natural ability. It's his supernatural work ethic that made him so good"? Is the secret this simple? Hard work?

Absolutely! The foundation of confidence is neither glamorous nor mysterious. It's boring, grueling, dirty, and monotonous. It hurts and it's very lonely. It requires constant sacrifice. It's rarely fun. *If you want to feel like a champion, then start training like one*. Your secret to success and building confidence is a four letter word: *WORK*. The mental state of trust in one's self that we're calling self-confidence comes *mainly* from your physical preparation. How you practice and "pay your physical dues" ultimately determines how confident you'll feel when you compete.

> **I**f you want to feel like a champion, start training like one.

Russia's Alexander Korellin demonstrates this secret better than most. Korellin is probably one of the greatest Greco-Roman wrestlers in the history of the sport. He is *unbeaten in international competition* and has won six world championships and three Olympic gold medals (1988, 1992, 1996). Despite the fact that Korellin has never failed a drug test in his life, his critics have long accused him of using performance-enhancing drugs. A proud and tremendously confident champion, Korellin patiently points out that the secret to his success lies not in drugs, but in the extreme intensity of his training. "I train like a madman . . . let my critics try that . . . those who accuse me have never trained one day in their life the way that I train each and every day of mine."

Korellin's words are indeed the secret to developing confidence and mental toughness as an athlete. This is not to say that your mental strategies (Step 2) can't bolster or undercut your confidence. Your self-talk and focus of concentration can have a significant impact on how you feel about yourself and can sometimes transcend your physical training. However, if you really want to build confidence, you must start with the foundation—your physical preparation. You can't develop the mind-set of a champion by cutting corners in training.

For example, a roller skater I'd been working with was about to compete in regionals to qualify for nationals. Alice had developed a lot of mental skills through our sessions and was confident that she'd be able to stay focused, handle the pressure, and move on to her next goal of placing at nationals. Regionals, however, turned out to be a disaster for Alice. She "popped" her jumps, doing singles where doubles were supposed to be, and fell several times. Her spins weren't sharp and she seemed to lack the energy and endurance necessary to rise to the challenge of this big competition. Not only was she beaten by skaters with far less talent, but she failed to qualify for nationals.

When Alice explained her poor performance to me, she claimed that she had choked, that it was all in her head. She went on to say that for some reason, when she stepped out to skate, she just lost her confidence. When I talked to her coach, she confirmed that confidence was a big part of the issue. She agreed that being unsure of herself greatly contributed to Alice's poor skating. However, she was convinced the girl hadn't choked and instead felt that her lack of confidence was related to her training.

According to her coach, Alice's meltdown was a direct result of an unwillingness to work hard. For the two weeks leading up to regionals, the biggest competition of the year, the skater only went to *half* the scheduled practices. When she was on the floor, she was working at about 20 percent efficiency, socializing with the boys and generally being distracted. The frustrating thing for the coach was that Alice's lack of serious effort had been going on for several years. The coach summed up the situation: "It's very simple the way I see it. Alice has the potential to become a champion. I don't mean to win regionals or even nationals. I mean, she has the talent to become a *world champion!* I've coached over 35 years and trust me, she's got it. However, she doesn't do anything with it. She's not working. She hasn't worked one day for me in four years! *How can you possibly have any confidence in yourself when you haven't been doing what you need to do?*"

Alice's coach was right. Confidence comes directly from proper physical and mental preparation. The only way to be fully prepared is by correctly practicing something over and over again until you can execute it without thinking. In Step 1 of the slump-busting model, "Ruling Out Nonmental Causes," I stated that not all performance slumps are in your head. Slumps can be directly caused by weaknesses in the physical, tactical, or technical parts of your sport. Alice's low confidence stemmed from a lack of physical endurance and technical expertise, both a result of a repeated failure to train adequately. Confidence comes from being able to answer honestly the two questions that Howard Ferguson, author of *The Edge*, asked his wrestlers daily: "Am I doing the very best I possibly can? Am I doing it every day?"[1]

There are no painless shortcuts for developing self-confidence. There is no handy pill you can swallow three times daily to get it into your system. Neither confidence nor success happen overnight while you sleep. The fastest way to get there is quite slow. The secret is simultaneously easy and hard. It's available to everyone, but precious few will actually use it. Preparation and practice. Pure, unadulterated hard work. Pushing yourself to the limit. As Korellin put it, "I train like a madman." Doing whatever it takes today and then dragging that tired, sore body out of bed and doing it again tomorrow, and the next day.

Confidence comes directly from proper physical and mental preparation.

Confidence means feeling like a winner. However, you can't expect to feel like a winner unless you can *physically* prove to yourself that you have the capability to become one. This physical proof has to come the old-fashioned way. Like Alexander Korellin, you have to earn it, day after day, week after week, month after month, year after year.

Feeling confident takes sticking to physical and technical basics. You must learn the fundamentals of your sport and then overlearn them. This solid foundation of proper fundamentals allows you to improvise later, when you get better.

When tennis pro Jimmy Connors first broke onto the international scene, he popularized the metal racket, blistering strokes, a signature two-handed backhand, and a hot temper. Soon everyone was wearing his clothing line, using his rackets, hitting a two-handed backhand, and using obscene gestures on the court. At the time, I was teaching tennis full time. One day a new pupil arrived early for his lesson. He looked like a Jimmy Connors clone. He wore a headband and wristlets just like Connors, was dressed in matching Connors-endorsed shirt and shorts, and had two of Jimmy's autographed metal rackets. Not only did he hit his backhand with two hands, but he made rude comments on the court, just like Connors. I was delighted at my good fortune. I excitedly began to plan my early retirement, thinking about all the money I could make as his coach and agent on the pro tour.

As I started to hit this 12-year-old a few balls to see what real skills he had, I was shaken out of my reverie by a Connors-like forehand drive that almost took my head off. When the second shot was harder than the first, I suggested that perhaps he might want to swing just a little slower. His third swing, a backhand, was just as hard as the first two, and the ball wedged itself into the back fence. From then on, things went from hard to harder. He spent the entire lesson pounding the ball with strokes that were a teaching pro's nightmare. No matter how many times or ways I suggested he slow his strokes down, he continued to swing away. After all, when you're Jimmy Connors, you crush the ball. What did I know anyway?

What young "Jimmy" didn't understand was that before you can hit that hard with control, you have to learn how to hit with proper form and the correct fundamentals. You can't derive real confidence from external trappings. Looking a certain way may fool your opponents for a few minutes, but ultimately they will catch on to the ruse. Even more important, you won't be able to fool yourself. Further, confidence is about staying within yourself when you perform and doing what *you* know how to do best. It's about playing your *own* game and not trying to be someone else or do what others are doing. It's about sticking to *your* game plan and competing the same way that you practiced.

Primarily, however, self-confidence comes from the knowledge that you've put at least as much effort into your training as everyone else. Look for opportunities to practice "the little differences that make a difference." What can you do in practice today that will give you a slight edge over your competition? Will you train 15 minutes longer? Will you deliberately go harder? At the end of practice, will you drive yourself to put everything you have into the final wind sprints? Will you run one more mile than everyone else or do 15 more push-ups? College coach and legendary wrestler Dan Gable motivated himself to train hard by imagining his Russian competition working out intensively at the moment. When Gable finished his workout and imagined his competitor also finishing and heading to the shower, Gable continued his session, doubling his training efforts for an additional few minutes.

Former NFL quarterback Roger Staubach summed up the key to developing winning self-confidence: "Confidence comes from hours and days and weeks and years of constant work and dedication. When I'm in the last two minutes of a December playoff game, I'm drawing confidence from wind sprints I did the previous March. It's just a circle; work and confidence, then more work and more confidence."[2]

What Staubach is saying is very basic. You build self-confidence by understanding that it is a privilege, not a right. You *earn* the privilege to trust yourself by what you do *today* and *every day* in practice.

Take Responsibility for Your Training

Some athletes talk a good game. Their confidence comes only from their lips. These athletes *seem* to exude confidence and won't hesitate to tell you or anyone who'll listen how great they are. Interestingly, when these athletes fail, their confident bravado continues as they offer numerous excuses

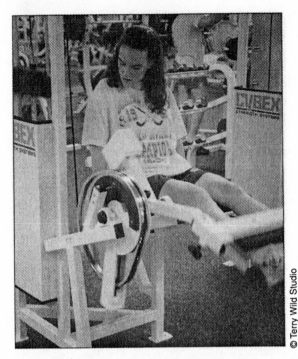

© Terry Wild Studio

for the failure, none of which have to do with *them*. They explain to whomever will listen that it just wasn't their fault. After all, it was really too cold to play well, the field should have been condemned by the Board of Health, the officiating was terrible, and the opponents cheated.

Talk, however, is cheap. If you have to tell people how good you are, then chances are you don't really believe it yourself. If you're constantly making excuses and blaming others for your setbacks, then deep down, you're loaded with self-doubts. Confidence is about action, not talk. When you talk up yourself or blame others, you're just masking your own insecurities. Confidence is powerfully quiet and speaks through actions and results, not empty words. In this way, confidence is about taking responsibility for your training. It's about putting your efforts and actions where your mouth is.

Think about U for a moment. I don't mean Y.O.U., but the letter "U." Every time you work out, your training efforts go into your U (see figure 8.1). If the quality and intensity of your training is good, then you're putting a lot of good stuff into U. You are taking the right fork toward success, as we discussed in Step 7 (see figure 7.1). If you blow off practice, back down when you're tired, or regularly take mental vacations during your sessions (the left fork on the road to mediocrity), then you are putting a significant amount of nothing or garbage into U.

Sooner or later all athletes come up against a situation in which their backs are to the wall and the pressure is cranked up to the max. It could be bases loaded, two outs, bottom of the ninth, with your team facing elimination when you step to the plate. Your previous two at-bats were unproductive, yet everyone is still depending on you. Perhaps you're the only defender between your opponent and the goal line, he's twice as big as you are, and you've got to stop him to save the game. Maybe it's the last mile of the marathon, you're running on empty, and your archrival just blew by you. Now you must make your move.

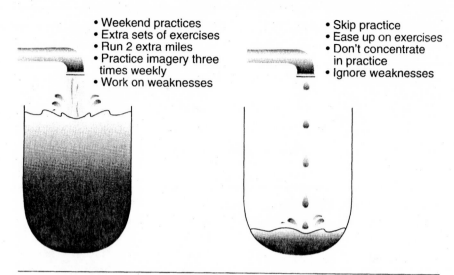

• Weekend practices
• Extra sets of exercises
• Run 2 extra miles
• Practice imagery three
  times weekly
• Work on weaknesses

• Skip practice
• Ease up on exercises
• Don't concentrate
  in practice
• Ignore weaknesses

Figure 8.1 What are you putting into U?

During these emotionally and physically trying times, you must dig deep inside yourself and come up with what you're really made of. What you're "really made of" is exactly what you've been putting into that U over the past days, weeks, months, and years. If you haven't put much in there because of continually taking the wrong road at the fork, then you're going to come up confidence-less and empty-handed, like Alice, the roller skater. If you've been putting garbage in there, then that's exactly what you'll pull up. However, if you've been conscientiously taking the right road and filling that U with consistency, gutsiness, dedication, determination, extra work, and a positive attitude, then you'll come up with the confidence to produce a winning effort. It's really a very simple, yet powerful formula. *No deposit, no return.*

In the 1996 U.S. Olympic Trials, the women gymnasts were competing for only five available spots because injured gymnasts Shannon Miller and Dominique Moceanu had been given passes onto the team, based on the strength of their previous performances at nationals. The competition was tight. Amy Chow was on the balance beam, one of the last events. In the middle of her routine, she slipped and fell, smashing her face into the side of the beam just below her left eye. She was clearly hurt and shaken up by the fall. However, without hesitation she got back up and not only completed her routine, but confidently stuck several difficult moves in the process. Her gutsy recovery landed her a place on the Olympic squad. We don't have to wonder what she had been consistently putting into her U.

So what kind of investment are you willing to make in your future? If you *really* want to feel winning confidence, what are you going to deposit in your U *today?* Will you take responsibility for your training? When the coach leaves you alone for an hour or two, will you pick up the intensity of your training or pick up the suntan lotion? When practice is canceled because the field is flooded, will you cheer all the way to the video arcade, or will you head indoors to run sprints and lift weights? Will you live the creed "If it is to be, it is up to me" or "If there's an easy way out, I'm there"?

> **Y**ou, above everyone else, are ultimately responsible for your success or failure.

You, above everyone else, are ultimately responsible for your success or failure. You don't grow true confidence by cruising down the road to mediocrity and making excuses. Further, you don't build confidence or mental toughness by blaming others. That kind of behavior simply prevents you from moving forward toward your goals. Nor can you feel that inner sense of trust if you depend on others to make things happen for you. Confidence emerges from consistently taking charge of the elements in your training environment that you can control, taking the initiative when others don't, being dissatisfied with mediocre efforts, and not colluding with those who look for the easy way out. "If it is to be" is truly up to *you*. Are you doing everything in your power to make that dream a reality?

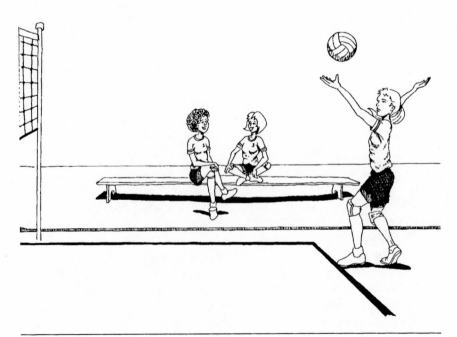

Take responsibility for your training.

Strengthen Your Weaknesses

Developing confidence in yourself also comes from the proper *follow-through*. You can't consistently hit that three-point shot without the correct follow-through. Without the right follow-through in swimming, your stroke shortens and you slow down. In almost every sport, your performance mechanics and control break down without a correct follow-through. Similarly, you can't become a confident champion without following through in *all* aspects of your daily training. The physical and emotional follow-through on your commitment to your goals and personal excellence helps you build a solid base of confidence.

An important, confidence-building aspect of this follow-through is how you choose to work on your weaknesses in the sport. If there's one thing that isn't fun, it's practicing your weak skills. When you begin to work on any weakness, you experience a minicrisis of confidence. It doesn't feel good to do things that you do poorly. It's far easier and much more fun to practice your strengths. Having to face your weaknesses usually makes you feel inadequate. When I coached tennis, I'd see this problem a great deal. For example, a player would do everything in his power to avoid working on his backhand. He'd spend three extra hours hitting serves, run more laps, endlessly repeat a forehand drill, and even *do his homework* before he would work on that dreaded backhand.

However, a chain is only as strong as its weakest link. Your game is limited most by your weaknesses. This weak link in your chain will ultimately undermine your confidence. If you never practice that backhand, you can't feel confident when your opponent pounds away at it. Even if you can avoid these weaknesses, sooner or later they'll catch up to you. Running around the backhand every chance you get won't take you to the next level. Facing your weaknesses and honestly working on them will. Working on your weaknesses is a powerful way to bust a slump, improve your overall performance, and build the confidence that fuels mental toughness.

Y*our game is limited most by your weaknesses.*

Colorado Rockies second baseman Eric Young is a classic example of this concept. In 1995, he led the National League in errors at his position, wouldn't get his body in front of the ball, and was clumsy around the bag on double plays. In 1996 spring training, he was forced to avoid his strength, hitting, and work exclusively on his fielding because of a fractured right hand. For the first few weeks of training, he couldn't even throw a ball, so instead, he practiced working on his weakness by fielding 500 grounders a day. The change, although predictable, has been amazing. Through 55 games, he had committed only one error and was much better at double plays. His bad break turned out to be just the break he needed to improve his game and increase his confidence.

Make a commitment to yourself *today* to spend more time identifying and strengthening your weak links. You don't have to enjoy the process. Few do at first. Understand, however, that working on your weaknesses is one more important way of *getting comfortable being uncomfortable*, so that you can bust your slump and become a champion. Many athletes you face make a science of avoiding their weaknesses. They prefer to stay in their comfort zone. By consistently stepping outside of yours and working on your shortcomings, you'll be developing a competitive advantage over them.

Set Up Your Training Environment to Boost Self-Confidence

Confidence grows by consistently training hard, using proper mechanics, and following through on the commitment that you make to yourself. In short, by *what* and *how much* you deposit in your account. Whether you follow through or not largely depends on *remembering what to do* and *being motivated to do it*. Knowing what to do by itself will not help you become a champion. You must also feel *compelled* to do it every day. By deliberately setting up your training environment in a certain way, you can insure that you remember what to do and feel the immediacy to then do it.

> **S**et up your training environment with reminders
> that will help you stay focused and create the
> immediacy you need to get the job done.

Set up your training environment with reminders that will help you stay focused and will create the immediacy you need to get the job done. A common example is having your written goals and big-enough why posted where you can easily see them many times a day (see Step 7). If you've taped your goals on the ceiling over your bed, they become the last thing that you see before you go to bed at night and the first thing that you see when you wake up. Whenever I sit down at my computer, whether I'm writing, surfing the Net, or attempting to avoid reality, I have to face a sign that reminds me, in big bold letters, of an important project I *really* want to accomplish. Immediately next to that sign is a question similarly posted at eye

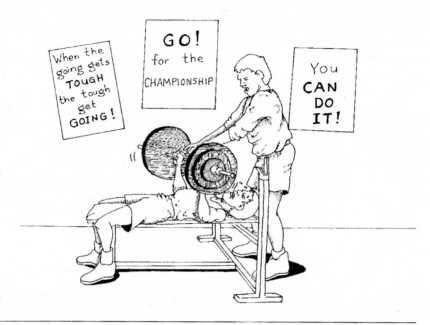

Set up your training environment for success.

level: "Are your actions right now goal-achieving or tension-relieving?" Much as I'd like to play another game of computer solitaire, these reminders motivate me to stay on task.

Many college and professional teams take advantage of negative press by posting these stories around the locker room. Looking at the derogatory comments of opposing teams or coaches serves as a daily source of motivation for these athletes to train harder. For example, during the 1996 NBA season, Chicago Bulls star Michael Jordan was upset by a negative comment that Seattle Sonics player Gary Payton made to the press about Jordan's skills. Payton claimed that Jordan was overrated and that he could be contained. Jordan was determined to make Payton pay for his remarks. Unfortunately, however, the Bulls were not scheduled to play the Sonics for almost three months. Jordan cut out the article, made several copies, and gave one to the team trainer. He instructed the trainer to show him the article a few days before their next Seattle game. Jordan set up his environment in this way so that he could *remember* what he wanted to do. Seeing the article again would then *motivate* him to follow through on his promise to himself.

Anson Dorrance, the head women's soccer coach at the University of North Carolina, is a master of setting up the training environment to foster intensity, develop confidence, and fuel motivation. Dorrance's record,

348-10-10 and 12 NCAA championships, speaks to his effectiveness with this strategy. In his program, Coach Dorrance creates what he calls a "competitive cauldron" in the team's daily training and match schedule.[3] The Lady Tar Heels' game schedule is designed to be difficult and regularly pits them against the best teams in the country. As a coach, if you want to consistently build confidence in your athletes, getting them comfortable being uncomfortable with tough opponents will help. Former University of Massachusetts men's basketball coach John Calipari used this strategy in transforming the Minutemen from cellar-dwellers into one of the top college teams in the country. However, constantly putting a team up against better teams could backfire; uninterrupted defeat won't boost anyone's confidence. Coaches should challenge their players by giving them the best competition possible.

In practice, coach Dorrance's competitive cauldron is even more intense. He has his players continually competing against each other in every aspect of their training, from conditioning and skill execution to scrimmaging. Results of all these minicompetitions are posted daily throughout the year, so that players always know where they stand. According to Dorrance, the kind of player who wants to be a champion will fight to the top of these ladders. If a player is not invested in this pursuit of excellence, her ranking won't matter.

In the book *Training Soccer Champions*, former North Carolina player Rosalind Santana discussed the effects of Dorrance's competitive cauldron on developing her self-confidence. "People are amazed at how I'll never settle for second best. I got that mentality here. We never entered a season thinking that maybe we'll take second this year. We always approached it like, 'Are we going to be national champions or not?' But the extra edge we have in practice is what's important. Almost everything we do in practice is recorded, and every week we got to see where we stand. And who wants to be at the bottom of the list?"[4] This daily knowledge that, as an athlete, you have done everything you possibly can and have trained harder than most will infuse in you a healthy dose of confidence.

By following the lead of coaches like Anson Dorrance or John Calipari, you can help your team develop the confidence of a champion. Structure your practices so that your players get comfortable being uncomfortable. Help them build a base of solid fundamentals. Teach them how to use superior conditioning as a competitive edge, so that they daily look for that little difference that will make a difference. Teach them to take responsibility for their training and encourage them to work on strengthening their weaknesses. Few athletes are self-driven enough to push themselves this hard. Most need you to structure the training environment to encourage them to go beyond their perceived limits. By helping them do this, you'll build a confidence in your players that is unstoppable.

Additional Confidence-Building Strategies

What else can you do to further develop your self-confidence and build mental toughness? Use the following strategies to add muscle to your self-confidence and push that slump farther into the background.

Use Your Weaknesses as Strengths

Swimmer Tom Dolan views the fact that he has only 20 percent of the lung capacity of his competitors as an advantage. He claims that because of this disability, he has had to work much harder and be mentally tougher than everyone else. The pain that he has to endure in training is much more severe than that endured by a normal swimmer. Consequently, he has learned how to master it. Since excellence in swimming is largely based on how well you can psychologically handle the pain and fatigue of oxygen deprivation, Dolan is getting better practice in this aspect than his competition. Similarly, wrestling great Dan Gable seriously injured his knee while training for the 1972 Olympics. Gable continued his training using just one leg. He claimed that learning how to wrestle on one leg made him a smarter, better wrestler. Sometimes your greatest handicaps can become your greatest strengths. Get in the habit of looking at your liabilities as assets.

Remind Yourself That You've Paid Your Dues

Remind yourself every chance you get of what you've put into your training. Keep close to the front of your mind all those sacrifices, the two-a-days, and the extra sessions. It's easy to forget how well-prepared you are when you're under the stress of a big competition. Before a competition, mentally review your training efforts and then tell yourself over and over that you're ready, that you've done what it takes to be the best. Focus on what you've done to prepare, not on what you haven't done.

Catch Yourself Doing Things Right

Keep track of all the gains you've made in your journey toward your ultimate goal. One way to do this and reinforce your confidence is to regularly maintain a "victory log." This log is a performance and training journal in which you post small victories that you achieve from practice and competition. Going an extra 10 minutes, pushing through a fatigue barrier when you wanted to quit, reaching a minigoal, getting a hit, a coach's positive comment, or winning a drill in practice should all be recorded in your log. When you catch yourself doing things right, you'll build confidence. Carry your log with you as part of your everyday equipment and review it the night before and day of a practice or competition.

Work With a Coach Who Believes in You

Picking the right kind of coach is one way of setting up your environment to remind and motivate you. Nothing can strengthen your confidence "muscle" quite like being with a coach who believes in your potential and encourages you. Whereas excessive, even well-meaning negativity undercuts confidence, a positive coach solidifies your trust in yourself. Besides yourself, your coach is probably the most important member of your team. Choose this teammate wisely. Having the knowledge and experience to help you become a champion will be of no help if the coach robs you of your self-confidence.

Twenty-one year old professional golfing sensation Tiger Woods can teach anyone a little something about developing slump-busting confidence. On April 13, 1997, Woods stunned the golf world by obliterating the field in The Masters, his first major tournament as a professional, to effortlessly win by 12 shots. Along the way he set a course record of 270, the lowest score in tournament history, and became the youngest man by two years to win at Augusta National Golf Club.

Woods demonstrated an unwavering confidence, nerves of steel, and extraordinary focus as he played a game that seemed well beyond that of a normal 21-year-old. Even when Masters officials gave him a warning for slow play on the tournament's second day, Woods kept his cool. How did he develop this kind of winning composure and self-assurance?

From the time he was 6 years old, Tiger started building his mental game with the help (not pushing) of his father, Earl Woods. He began listening to subliminal tapes with messages of belief, focus, and confidence (such as "I believe in me," "I will my own destiny,"

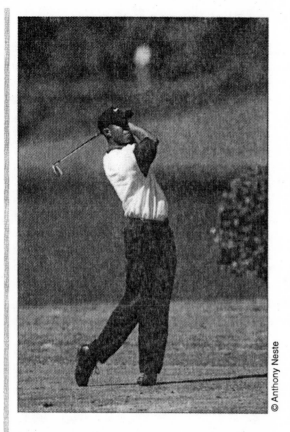

© Anthony Neste

and "I smile at obstacles"). He made signs displaying the messages in these tapes and posted them all around his room. When Tiger was 7, Earl began to teach him to expect the best and prepare for the worst by creating obstacles and distractions while Tiger was swinging or putting.[5] Soon none of his father's deliberate psychological warfare had any impact on him.

Earl instilled in his son a pure love for the game that seemed to help him transcend normal performance problems. Tiger played because of this passion and seemed oblivious to fear of mistakes and failures. Neither his self-esteem nor his ego seemed to be in danger when he stepped up to the tee. His love for the game drove him to practice long and hard, regardless of the weather or playing conditions. In many ways this work ethic has greatly enhanced his self-confidence. His coach, Butch Harmon, claimed that Tiger wanted to work with him 24 hours a day.[6]

When he was 13, Woods worked with a sports psychologist who taught him how to use hypnosis and trance to further block out conscious mind interference and strengthen his resolve and focus. His skills in hypnosis helped him go to such deep levels of concentration that he couldn't even remember making certain shots.

Tiger's phenomenal success is a product of the fine blending of well-developed physical and mental skills with a tremendous passion and work ethic. He claims that he wants to be the best golfer ever, and in many ways he's already started to prove that he will be.[7]

Feed Yourself High-Confidence Food

If you're in training and eat foods high in sugar or fat, you'll feel lousy and your resultant low energy level will adversely affect your performance. As they say in the computer world, "garbage in, garbage out." The converse of this is also true: "good stuff in, good stuff out." Similarly, your mental diet can dramatically affect your self-confidence. By feeding yourself material that is "high in confidence" from books, audiotapes, and videotapes, you can bolster your self-confidence. Reading nonfiction about individuals in and out of sports who've successfully pursued their dreams against all odds (*I Never Had It Made* by Jackie Robinson; *The Four-Minute Mile* by Roger Bannister; *Live Your Dreams* by Les Brown; and biographies of Winston Churchill, Abraham Lincoln, Martina Navratilova, and Amelia Earhart), will help you stay on the right path. Listening to and watching motivational and training tapes will inspire you and foster that all-important inner trust. For example, movies like "Hoosiers," "Rudy," and "Chariots of Fire" are not only inspirational, but are also based on true stories.

Develop a Confidence-Enhancing Nickname

Having a special identity can help you reach beyond yourself to peak performance. For example, Pete's tennis coach would affectionately call him "Pancho" after the legendary touring great Pancho Gonzales. At first, there was nothing Pancho-like about Pete's game. Pete was an average player. He told me, however, that the nickname made him feel special and inspired him to work harder. Soon his play began to reflect the work and the nickname. If a coach is sincere in the use of such a nickname, it can help an athlete or team develop a special identity that serves as a continuous confidence-booster.

Develop and Use Rituals

Going into competition, your rituals can help you stay calm and feel good about yourself. In Step 3 we discussed the importance of using preperformance rituals to help you control your concentration the minutes leading up to the start. Rituals begun the night before and day of the contest can also keep your confidence high. Whether it's a ritual your team uses on an away bus trip, a certain pregame meal, or a special song that you play to yourself, repeating a familiar routine will help you maintain that all-important trust in yourself. The familiar always neutralizes fear and bolsters self-confidence. Rituals are yet another way that you can gain some control over your environment.

Conclusion

Learning to exercise and strengthen your "confidence muscle" will take you one step closer to busting that slump and performing to your potential. Self-confidence is one of those trademarks of the mentally tough athlete. Your trust in yourself gives you the courage to take the risks necessary to become a champion, and your ability to take risks is largely determined by how well you handle setbacks.

Confident athletes view failures and setbacks differently than do most people. Their sense of personal control and belief in themselves are not significantly shaken by these disappointments. Deep down they remain confident that they will ultimately prevail, and this confidence keeps them moving forward. Mentally tough athletes use their confidence to pick themselves up and keep going after each fall. Their persistence and ability to rebound in the face of repeated failures lead them to success time and time again.

In the next step of the slump-busting model, you will learn how to use your self-confidence to master the skill of reboundability and use it to turn yourself into a model of mental toughness. As you learn how to move beyond failures and adversity, your mental toughness will grow.

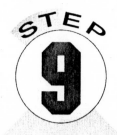

BECOMING
MENTALLY TOUGH

"Failure is the perfect stepping stone to success."

Mental toughness is the ability to stand tall in the face of adversity. It's a psychic resiliency that allows you to rebound from setbacks and failures time and time again. Mental toughness is the attitude my martial arts teacher expressed this way: "If you get knocked down once, you get up once. If you get knocked down twice, you get up twice. But if you get knocked down eight times, get up nine!"

> **M**ental toughness is the outward manifestation
> of an inner commitment.

Mental toughness is the outward manifestation of an inner commitment. It's a refusal to quit on that dream, no matter what. It's the child's inflatable punching doll that keeps bouncing back up, regardless of how hard you pound it. Mental toughness seems to defy reality and sometimes even common sense. It propels athletes forward against staggering odds, enabling them to find the possible in the impossible.

The Stuff of Mental Toughness

Like self-confidence, mental toughness is a "psychological muscle" that is frequently underdeveloped in the slumping athlete. With the proper "exercise," however, you can learn to build this muscle until it becomes one of your primary strengths. The next step in our slump-busting model is to develop the mental toughness of a champion. Of all the physical and mental assets an athlete has, mental toughness is by far the most important. Without the ability to keep bouncing back up, all of your other efforts, skills, and talents become useless.

> **O**f all the physical and mental assets an athlete has, mental toughness is by far the most important.

Anybody can act, think, and feel tough when the sun is shining and the temperatures are pleasant. When everything in your life and training is going your way, it's easy to feel like a winner. Keeping yourself motivated under these conditions is easy. Precious few individuals, however, can maintain this same sunny disposition when the skies turn dark and a twister lays waste to all that they've worked hard to build. It's during these bleak times that the athlete's character is put to the true test.

1996 Olympic double gold-medal sprinting sensation Michael Johnson tested his mental toughness in 1992 in Barcelona, Spain. A sure bet for a gold medal in the 200, Johnson came down with food poisoning several weeks before the Olympics and finished a devastating fourth. His ability to bounce back and do what no man had ever done before, win gold in both the 200 and 400, was powered by his mental toughness.

From a life perspective, however, Johnson's adversity pales in comparison to Cuban runner Ana Quirot's trials. A world-class athlete, model, and national treasure, Quirot won gold in Barcelona. Two years later, while working over a kerosene stove, she was badly burned over 40 percent of her body when the stove exploded. Pregnant at the time, Quirot lost her baby and almost her life. She fought back and, against all odds, began training again. In 1995 she won a silver medal in the 800-meter run at the World Championships. In the Atlanta Olympic Games in 1996, she again won silver in that event. What enabled her to pick up the shattered pieces of her life and go on? Mental toughness.

Where does this precious commodity come from? The success of Chinese female athletes, long dominant on the world's stage, might provide us with some important clues. First, Chinese women regularly train with the men. This stiffer competition is certainly part of the answer. Constantly going up against stronger training partners will push your limits, build confidence, and make you tougher. As we discussed in Step 8, this is a great way to train yourself to get comfortable being uncomfortable. In addition to tough training competition, the Chinese women athletes sometimes had to withstand punishing and abusive workout regimes imposed by their coaches. When you live in an abusive, deprived environment, everything else you face seems mild by comparison.

The overall key to Chinese dominance may lie in the phrase *chi ku*, which means to *eat bitterness*. According to Tian Wenhui, the head of the committee governing the network of specialty schools that produce roughly 95 percent of the country's elite athletes, "Chinese women are better able to eat bitterness and endure hardship than Western women."[1] They have more practice at eating bitterness in their day-to-day lives and training than most other athletes.

There's no question that setbacks, deprivation, and hardship make a person tougher. Athletes who have things go their way all the time are vulnerable and ultimately weak. How can they possibly be prepared to deal with disappointment if they never practice it? Without experiencing adversity themselves, how can they understand that failures and setbacks are a normal part of the process of reaching their goals?

Many young athletes who experience nothing but success early in their careers end up prematurely quitting their sport when they start to run into roadblocks. Blessed by early developmental advantages, these athletes breeze through the competition, enjoying size, strength, speed, and skill advantages. During adolescence, however, their competition begins to catch up developmentally. Soon these athletes are being challenged and beaten by opponents that they've long dominated. Having never learned to work harder and persevere in the face of hardship, they become too easily discouraged. Rather than tough it out, they mistakenly believe they no longer have what it takes to be a winner, and give up.

The lesson here is quite simple, yet critically important. To *really* enjoy the sweet taste of victory, you have to eat your share of bitterness. If you are struggling with a slump, know that your difficulties ultimately will make you mentally tougher than someone who has never had to endure these same frustrations.

Mastering Failure

The key to developing mental toughness is learning how to handle failure and to put it to work for you. Schools today often don't teach the value of failing. How many times has a teacher told you, "You learn from your mistakes"? While this statement is true, the underlying message communicated in most classrooms is that failure is a bad thing, a cause for humiliation, and therefore something to be avoided. When a child answers a question incorrectly, "he's stupid" is an unexpressed response from many classmates. When graded tests are handed back, students who scored low feel embarrassed or inadequate, *not* as if they are having a *learning experience*. It's a rare teacher or coach today who can genuinely communicate that failure and making mistakes are an integral and critically important part of learning.

Recently I got a call from a 13-year-old gymnast who was stuck on a number of skills involving moving backward. Her repeated failures to master these skills had driven her impatient coach to publicly poke fun at her, leaving this gymnast feeling ashamed about her difficulties. In the process, the coach unknowingly communicated a very unhelpful message to all the other gymnasts present: "Getting stuck, messing up, and failing are unacceptable in this gym and will get you humiliated."

Teaching athletes that they shouldn't make mistakes not only interferes with the learning process, but also violates a number of the principles of peak performance we discussed in the Introduction. When these principles are violated by coaches, athletes, and parents, performance problems *always* result. Fear of messing up creates performers who are tentative and cautious. It stops them from relaxing and taking risks (Principle #7). It puts the athletes in their head (Principle #6), and leads to choking. It distracts the athletes' focus from the process to the outcome (Principle #3). Fear of failure (Principle #4) is probably the biggest cause of choking. Furthermore, fear of failure and mistakes kills the athletes' enjoyment (Principle #1). When you teach athletes that making mistakes and failing is part of the process, you free them to give full, totally committed, and uninhibited effort.

You must take risks in life and in your sport to get the prize. The more risks you're willing to take, the more likely you'll be successful. Taking risks demands that you become oblivious to the possibility of failing. To win, you must learn to perform like you have nothing to lose. This is the ultimate paradox in sports and life. The secret to success is in failing. The key to winning is in losing. Focus too much on winning and you will lose. Block out winning from your consciousness and it will be waiting for you at the finish line. You can only win when you've accepted the possibility of failure and dismissed it from your mind. Failure is truly the perfect stepping stone to success.

While slumping athletes interpret setbacks and failures as a detour off the road to success, mentally tough competitors view these difficulties as part of the road leading to their goals. In the mind of mentally tough athletes, the rough spots are really no different from the smooth parts. You have to traverse both to reach your dreams.

> **Y**ou can only win when you've accepted the possibility of failure and dismissed it from your mind.

Perhaps handling failure is the one thing that winners do far better than losers. Those who "fail better" are more likely to reach their goals than those unskilled in mastering failure. The most powerful step you can take right now to develop mental toughness and put that slump behind you is to change how you handle your failures.

Handling failure does not mean that you must be satisfied with second best. Most committed athletes hate losing. The dissatisfaction with second place is most visible at high-level competitions like the Olympics. Olympic silver medalists often seem more disappointed by a second place finish than those winning bronze. The silver medalists expected gold and view the silver medal as a failure, while the third-place finishers are usually delighted just to have medalled.

Two behavior characteristics determine how you handle your failures: (1) your *perspective* or how you *view the failure* and (2) how you *explain the failure* to yourself. This is an artificial separation because these behaviors are interwoven. How you *view* your failure is affected by how you *explain* it to yourself, and how you *explain* it is colored by how you *view* it. However, for the purposes of our discussion and for providing intervention strategies, this separation will be useful.

Essentially, people use their failures in two main ways. Champions use failure as a valuable source of *feedback*. They get information that they need to learn how to get stronger, faster, smarter, and better. Their failures become a reason to recommit themselves to their goals and fuel their determination to succeed. Athletes lacking mental toughness, however, use their setbacks and failures as evidence of their inadequacy and worthlessness. They hold up their failures as proof of their incompetence. This use of failure demotivates the athletes and gives them a reason to abandon their quest.

Viewing Failure

How does a Tim Daggett (1984 gold medalist in gymnastics) come back from four *career-ending* injuries? How does a Dan Jansen (world record-holding speed skater) persevere through personal loss and multiple public failures to win gold? How does a track star like Gail Devers, critically ill and within a breath of having both legs amputated, return to health to claim the title of fastest woman alive? Their secret lies inside. A refusal to give up. A resilience. A certain perspective. Mental toughness.

Look at figure 9.1. Point B represents successful completion of your ultimate goal at some time in the future. Point A represents where you are today on that quest. As figure 9.1 depicts, there's a line that connects where you are today, point A, with your ultimate goal, point B. While there may be twists and turns in the actual road, the general direction, like climbing a mountain, is straight up.

If you've been stuck in a slump or blocked by fears, this graphic depiction of the road may strain the limits of your belief system. You can positively certify that there's nothing straight about this path. It's filled with wrong turns, dead ends, and athlete-eating potholes. Your slump or block is evidence of this.

Along this road are potholes like slumps and blocks that can indeed swallow you up for weeks and months at a time. You may even have other "opportunities" later on in your career to fall into another slump pothole. No need to panic at this thought. With the mental toughness you are developing, these athletic delays will most likely be less enduring than the one with which you're currently struggling.

Slumps and blocks, however, are not the only experiences that you'll encounter on your journey. You'll also experience moments of victory where you made the varsity, broke into the starting lineup, cleared five feet for the first time, broke that pesky time barrier, or were named as a high school All-American. "Getting there" is exciting and gratifying too.

As you continue upward toward your goal, don't forget all those experiences of getting cut, choking away the big match, failing to medal, sitting the bench, or tripping in the middle of the race. Remember also that no career is complete without a little sickness and a few injuries that force you to take an unwanted vacation. Then there are those plateaus or times when absolutely nothing seems to be happening. Not quite in a slump, but far from productive, you seem stalled along the side of the road while the rest of the competitive world seems to pass you by.

> **Y**ou always get closer to your goals after each
> bout with adversity.

While the road may appear straight in one direction, closer examination reveals all kinds of interesting peaks and valleys, starts and stops, broken pavement and smooth patches. Keeping this perspective of the *entire* path is critical to how well you will handle the adversity you are sure to encounter along the way. It's this perspective that will provide you with the will to keep going and underlies your developing mental toughness.

How can you remember to keep this perspective as you travel? By asking yourself the simple question, "With each failure and setback, am I getting closer to or farther away from my goals?" According to figure 9.1, the answer is clear. On this timeline *you* always *get closer to your goals after each bout with adversity.*

Since you can learn from your failures, these experiences actually provide more valuable information than your successes. Your breakdowns give

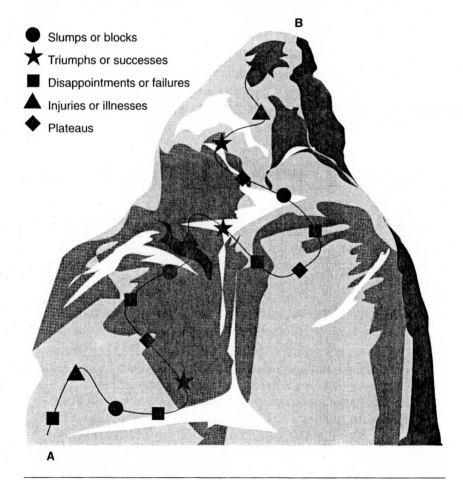

● Slumps or blocks
★ Triumphs or successes
■ Disappointments or failures
▲ Injuries or illnesses
◆ Plateaus

Figure 9.1 The road to success.

you immediate if not direct feedback as to what you're doing wrong and how you may correct the situation. Sometimes this information may be obscured by feelings of frustration and discouragement. However, with a little digging, you can easily uncover the important messages in the failure.

If keeping this long-term perspective of your journey is so critical to how you successfully handle failure, what else can you do to learn how to maintain such a perspective? The following exercise was designed to teach you how to view your setbacks and disappointments from a big-picture perspective. Practice this exercise to improve your reboundability from failure.

Regular practice of this exercise two or more times a week will help you change your perspective on the setbacks, hardships, and failures that are simply part of the normal scenery as you travel toward the realization of your ultimate goal. Viewing obstacles from this vantage point will increase your overall mental toughness, so that as you move through the rockier times, you will feel a resiliency and reboundability lacking in the slumping athlete. Just as important, mental toughness will help you manage the emotions of failure.

KNOWING THE ROAD

Do this exercise in an environment that's quiet and free from distractions. Allow approximately 10 to 15 minutes practice time. Recording the instructions on audiotape works the best. You can also read the instructions ahead of time and guide yourself through it. (Remember, if you do make a tape, speak slowly and pause several seconds when you see the series of dots [. . .].) Sit or lie comfortably and take a minute or two to relax yourself in any way that you'd like. Once you've begun to feel yourself slow down, proceed as follows:

Think about your ultimate goal for a moment. . . . Imagine that you have finally reached this milestone. . . . Perhaps you have just come back from the awards ceremony and you're at a party held in your honor. You can look around and see familiar faces . . . smiles. . . . Friends and family are offering words of praise, congratulatory hugs. . . . The party is in full swing, and you can begin to truly appreciate what you've actually accomplished. . . . Your dream has come true. . . . You may even find yourself signing autographs or talking to people you had only dreamed of meeting. . . . The champagne or soda pop may be flowing or you may be eating chocolate cake, because every great accomplishment deserves a celebration. . . .

And as you celebrate, sign autographs, or simply take in this wonderful moment, you find yourself moving off by yourself into a quiet room, removed from the crowd, to take a short break from the festivities. . . . You find a comfortable place to sit in this room and begin to think back . . . to all the situations, events, and hardships you went through over the last few years to get yourself here tonight to this celebration. . . . Starting with the most recent . . . you find yourself smiling again as you relive that crowning moment of glory, that ultimate performance . . . and then thinking back to everything in the recent past that prepared you for it . . . all the good training times and the bad . . . the things that were easy to swallow and those that left a bad taste in your mouth. . . .

And as you think back, you return to that last big setback . . . an injury, illness, disappointing performance, or simply a slump. . . . You may remember feelings of discouragement, depression . . . maybe even a desire to quit. . . . It is interesting that, as you celebrate tonight, you may even remember the times when you were close to packing it in. . . . And as you continue to think back . . . review the starts and stops . . . the highs and lows . . . going all the way back. . . . How many times were you just sure you were going to make it? . . . And all those times you were not so sure. . . .

Then there was that other big disappointment . . . that roadblock you thought you'd never get by. . . . How did you hang tough and persevere? . . . All of these moments can pass in front of your eyes right now as you review the path that you took . . . the coaches along the way . . . the one or two who believed in you and really made a difference in your life . . . the coaches you'd rather forget. . . . Go all the way back until that moment when the dream first began to crystallize in your mind. . . . Can you remember what it felt like when the path first popped into your head? . . . Perhaps you shared this dream and can recall now people's reactions . . . the support and encouragement . . . the laughs and ridicule. . . .

As you reflect back, you can truly appreciate the road that you chose . . . and how you stuck to it through all the good times and bad . . . and now you're finally here . . . you made it! . . . And you let your reflections slowly fade as you think about getting back to the party . . . have another piece of cake . . . sign a few more autographs . . . get a few more congratulatory hugs . . . and feel the emotions of a tremendous accomplishment. . . . And just note how your mental toughness propelled you through it all. . . . Then allowing that scene to slowly fade . . . let yourself return to this place and time.

Explaining Failure

If mastering hardships and failure were simply an intellectual process, you could stop reading here and, armed with your new perspective, instantly be transformed into Mr. or Ms. Mental Toughness. Unfortunately, adversity frequently bypasses your powers of logic, tapping directly into your emotions. Sometimes no matter how hard you try to think positively about a failure, your feelings become overwhelming. You tell yourself, "Losing is a learning experience" and "When you've put this slump behind you, you'll be stronger for it," but your emotions are speaking so loudly, you can't hear these words of reason.

How many times have you seen an athlete crash into the hard wall of failure and excitedly proclaim, "What a great learning experience!"? Can you imagine Greg Norman, in an interview after his dramatic, final-day collapse cost him the 1996 Masters, saying, "I'm so pleased that I've been given this opportunity to squander a six-stroke lead, totally humiliate myself in front of the world, and once again choke away another major tournament. I'm sure there's a very wonderful learning experience in all of this, and there are so many people I'd like to thank."

Failing is not something people enjoy, regardless of its value as a learning experience. Nor is failing something people do for recreation. You'd never hear a conversation like this: "Busy tonight, Billy? What say you and me go out and publicly embarrass ourselves, blowing our team's chances for the big championship?" "Great idea, Mikey, but only if I can be the real loser! You got to play that role last time. Now it's my turn." There's no question that while you go through this learning process, the emotions that arise from failing can be excruciating.

The Emotions of Failure. Your emotional reaction to failure can often blind your perspective and interfere with your ability to bounce back. While figure 9.1 clearly depicts that with each setback you actually get closer to the goal, the emotions attached to these experiences make you *feel* that the opposite is happening, that you're moving farther away. The emotions distort the process. They provide a narrow, close-up view of the failure that just happened and trick you into believing that this is the whole process.

> **Y**our emotional reaction to failure can often blind your perspective and interfere with your ability to bounce back.

Because of the power of your emotions to distort reality and knock you off track, how you handle these feelings is crucial to your ultimate success.

The story was heroic—the 1996 women's gymnastics team competition at the Atlanta Olympic Games. The climax, the stuff of a Rocky movie. The United States team was poised to win an unprecedented

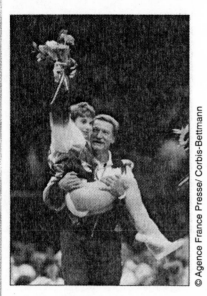

© Agence France Presse/ Corbis-Bettmann

gold medal and beat the legendary Romanians and the incomparable gymnasts of Russia. The vault was the last event and only two Americans remained, 14-year-old prodigy Dominique Moceanu and 18-year-old Olympic veteran Kerri Strug. The United States needed only one good vault to seal the win and put the gold medal out of reach of their competitors.

On the first of her two vaults, Moceanu sat down on her landing. She'd been nursing a hairline fracture in her leg and had been having this problem all week in practice. It was the only event that Dominique had been unable to regularly practice for the last month. Her second vault was an exact duplicate of the first. The crowd groaned and the tension mounted. Moceanu had just opened the door a crack for the competition. All eyes immediately turned to Strug, a Bela Karolyi pupil, who had labored in the shadows behind his 1992 superstar world champion, Kim Zmeskal, and who, since 1994, had taken a similar bridesmaid's role to Moceanu.

The mostly American crowd held its breath as Strug sprinted down the runway. She sprang off the board, flew through the air and landed awkwardly, her legs collapsing out from under her. Unlike Moceanu, however, Strug got up slowly and painfully—she injured her left ankle. She limped back as the cameras closed in on coach Bela Karolyi telling her to shake it off and trying to will her through the vault with his words, "You can do it . . . Yes, you can Kerri . . . You can do it." Strug headed to the top of the runway. She had lost feeling in the ankle and started rubbing it, then jogged in place, trying to keep it loose. Determination and pain were competing for expression on her face. Final vault. America's last chance to do the impossible. The door seemed to be opening wider for the Russians and Romanians. Strug began her approach, running at full throttle and blotting out the obvious discomfort. She nailed the vault and miraculously stuck her landing, grimacing painfully at the impact as the injured left foot hit the mat. She held that position on one foot, saluted the judges, and then collapsed in pain onto the mat. Her injury, torn ligaments, was severe enough to keep her out of the individual competitions. However, at this moment, it didn't matter. The United States women won their first team gold medal in gymnastics. Kerri Strug's gutsy performance lifted her to heroine status, and she was carried triumphantly out of the arena, her image soon to grace Wheaties boxes.

Strug's courageous display of grace under fire gave us a peek at the intensity that burns brightly within all great athletes. Strug had to have a special something to even find herself in this made-for-TV situation, let alone to come through a winner. Many others in her situation would have left the gym long before. To beat the hardships, disappointments, years of playing second fiddle, and a serious fall, Kerri had to be tough inside. She had to have abundant quantities of that priceless athletic commodity, *mental toughness.*

What are the emotions of failing? Disappointment. Anger. Discouragement. Self-doubts. Humiliation. Embarrassment. Sadness. Frustration. Shame. Hopelessness. Hopefulness. Determination. Feelings of inadequacy. When failure crosses the finish line first, some combination of these feelings will soon follow. Which ones you experience primarily depends upon how you *explain the failure to yourself.*

Explanatory Styles of Failure.   Baseball great Yogi Berra once claimed that he never blamed himself when he wasn't hitting. Instead, he blamed the bat, and if his hitting problems continued, he simply changed bats. In a similar way, Pete Rose felt that anytime he struck out, it was a fluke and nothing more. A local high school football coach, borrowing from a pro football coaching great, told me that his teams have never lost a game; they've merely run out of time. A professional tennis player of average ability informed me one day that when he walked out on the court, he always expected to play his best and win. If he didn't, he felt the other player had just gotten lucky that day.

Whenever you fail, you explain the failure to yourself. You may rationalize it away, blame your lack of ability, or simply attribute it to the astrological alignment of the sun, moon, and stars. Each of the aforementioned individuals explained their failures in a way that seemed to have no negative effect on their self-confidence. Contrast this with the swimmer who missed making an Olympic team in his event by .02 seconds and explained, "This kind of thing always seems to happen to me. I don't know why I still waste my time training . . . I don't think I have what it takes" or the star shooting guard who blew an uncontested seven footer that would have given her team the state championship and said, "I let the team down . . . I don't even deserve to be starting." These kinds of self-explanations for failing leave the athlete feeling worthless.

Your *explanatory style*, according to Martin Seligman, author of *Learned Optimism*, is the habitual way that you explain bad events to yourself.[2] It's more than just the words that you mouth when you fail, but your *habit of thought* learned in childhood and adolescence. Your explanatory style is critically important to your ultimate success or failure, because these explanations dramatically affect your motivation and persistence. For example, if you explain your failures the way the first group of athletes did, you're left feeling *optimistic* or hopeful. If you use explanations like the swimmer and basketball player, however, you're left feeling *pessimistic* or *hopeless*. Feelings of optimism are the hallmark of mental toughness and fuel a bull-dog determination. Pessimistic feelings, on the other hand, undercut your resiliency and determination to reach the goal. The swimmer and basketball player retired shortly after these failures.

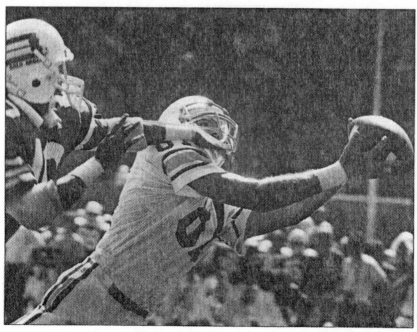

Y *our explanatory style dramatically affects*
your motivation and persistence.

How do you identify your current explanatory style? Seligman high-lights three crucial dimensions in how people explain their failures: *perma-nence, pervasiveness,* and *personalization.*

• **Permanence**—Mentally tough athletes who refuse to give up see ad-versity, losses, and setbacks as *temporary* events. The events happened once or twice, may even happen again, but they are *time-limited.* Athletes who easily give up view these same setbacks as *permanent.* They see their fail-ures in terms of "always" and their successes as "nevers" and "impossibles." Making statements to yourself about the never-changing quality of your failures (such as, "I'm a choker," "The coach never plays me," "I can't play ball to save myself," or "I always lose the important races.") throws up one more obstacle in your path to success. Instead, practice thinking about your abilities and failures in *temporary* terms, such as, "I haven't hit *lately*" and "*Sometimes* I get too nervous to perform well," not as permanent traits.

To master failure and develop mental toughness, you must learn how to view your setbacks, hardships, and personal shortcomings as temporary. Reserve permanent language for your strengths and successes (for example, "I always do well in the important races," "I never choke under pressure," or "I've got a good head on my shoulders."). Review Step 5, "Expecting Success," for further discussion and exercises on this topic.

• **Pervasiveness**—Some athletes come away from a bad performance and tell you *exactly* why they failed (for example, "I got a bad start," "My first service was inconsistent all match," "The refs made several bad calls today," or "I lost my shooting touch in the last quarter."). Each of these explanations is very *specific* and pinpoints the source of the problem. Other athletes, playing the same way, will explain their failures in more *general* terms (such as "My whole race was terrible," "I'm a weak tennis player," "All refs are blind and biased," or "I can't shoot to save my life."). The second group of explanations are *pervasive* and exaggerate the extent of the problem. It's as if there's a fire in a wastebasket, and someone tells the fire department that the whole house is burning to the ground.

While permanence refers to *time* in Seligman's model, pervasiveness is about *space.* Athletes who view their problems in this pervasive, all-encompassing way become easily discouraged and lose their motivation to persist. On the other hand, athletes who are able to limit their failures by explaining them in specific ways are more optimistic about a successful outcome and therefore more persistent. To develop into a mentally tough athlete, you must learn to view your failures and shortcomings in specific terms. Catastrophizing your setbacks will only undercut your confidence and drain your energies.

- **Personalization**—The final aspect of explanatory style, *personalization*, refers to your tendency to blame yourself *(internalize)* or blame others *(externalize)* for failures and bad events. When Yogi Berra says that it's the bat's fault if he's not hitting, he is *externalizing* the problem. When the tight end who drops the potential game-winning catch in the end zone says he has "stone fingers," he's *internalizing* the problem. If you're in the habit of blaming yourself every time you fail, you'll be left with no confidence and little motivation to succeed in the face of adversity. Externalizing your failures and setbacks, on the other hand, preserves your self-confidence and mental toughness.

When you lose and say *to yourself,* "I felt really terrible today," "The wind threw me off completely. . . . I could barely get my footing," or "I've been sick and that's why I faded big time at the end," you are placing the blame for your failure outside yourself. However, externalizing your failures does *not* mean that you can refuse to take responsibility for yourself and your training. "I didn't do the wind sprints today because the coach looked at me the wrong way," "We lost because the sun was shining too brightly," and "I didn't eat breakfast and the other team cheated" are all blatant examples of simply making excuses. As I mentioned in Step 9, your confidence comes directly from taking responsibility for yourself and your training. Winners do not look for excuses or point fingers. Externalizing failure is more of a *private* exercise that mentally tough athletes engage in to keep themselves moving toward their goals.

There is a big difference between taking responsibility for yourself and blaming yourself. Taking responsibility is a *constructive* process in which you seek to learn from your failures. Inherent in taking responsibility is a willingness to honestly examine yourself and your performance. Taking responsibility is solution-focused, in that the athletes acknowledge the problem and are willing to work to resolve it themselves.

Self-blame, on the other hand, is a useless and destructive process that stops once the athletes find the culprit (themselves) responsible for the failure. Instead of being solution-focused, it is problem-focused and therefore does not seek to strengthen weaknesses or correct flaws. It is an end unto itself. As a consequence, athletes who engage in self-blame are left feeling incompetent, weak, and hopeless.

In December of 1993, Bobby Hurley was on top of the world. A basketball sensation in college and four-year starter at point guard, he had led the Duke Blue Devils to back-to-back national championships in 1991 and 1992. He left college as a two-time first team All-American and the NCAA's all-time assist leader. He was the 7th pick overall in the 1993 NBA draft, chosen by the Sacramento Kings, who signed him to a six-year, $16.2 million contract.

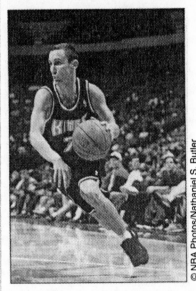

© NBA Photos/Nathaniel S. Butler

After he had played just 19 games, Hurley's NBA career was interrupted by an automobile accident that by all reports should have killed him. On the night of December 12th, while returning home after a game, Hurley's vehicle was struck broadside on the driver's side by a car traveling 55 miles per hour without its lights on. Wearing no seat belt, Hurley was thrown from the car and sustained severe injuries, including two collapsed lungs, a compression fracture in his lower back, and most serious of all, a torn trachea. According to the doctors who treated the basketball star, this injury results in death in more than 90 percent of such cases. Hurley also had five broken ribs, a shattered left shoulder blade, a torn anterior cruciate ligament in his right knee, a broken right fibula, multiple deep lacerations, and a badly sprained left wrist.

Eight hours of delicate surgery were required to reattach Hurley's trachea to his lung. That he survived at all was nothing short of miraculous—but that his basketball career was over was almost certain. In the two weeks following the accident, Hurley had to relearn how to open his eyes, sit up, and walk. His rehabilitation process was agonizing. Six weeks after the accident, having returned home to New Jersey, Hurley began going to a health club. At first, just the simple act of walking across the gym to a treadmill left him winded. His first attempt at sustained exercise was to walk a mile in 10 minutes.

By early March he was running, and in April he began to play games of one-on-one with a personal trainer. Hurley was determined and totally committed to playing again. Soon he was drilling hard for 75 minutes in addition to running, lifting weights, and doing sit-ups. He gained back all but 5 of the 20 pounds he had lost and accomplished what many thought to be impossible. When he returned to the Kings' preseason camp he was in the best shape of his life.

But poor shooting during the 94-95 season kept him on the bench, and his playing time dwindled. While he played in a career-high 72 games in the 95-96 season, he averaged less than 15 minutes per game, a career low.

Limited playing time continued to hamper Hurley's comeback bid until the Kings changed coaches in March 1997, replacing Gary St. Jean with Eddie Jordan. Jordan moved Hurley from the number three guard up to a starting position, and Bobby responded like the Hurley of old. In his April starts he averaged 28 minutes, 10 assists, and almost 7 points per game. Bobby Hurley refused to quit, and his guts, determination, and mental toughness helped him do the impossible.[3,4,5]

Onward to Mental Toughness

If your habitual way of explaining your failures has eroded your mental toughness, what can you do about it? Start by closely examining the dialogue of your inner coach for *permanent, pervasive,* and *personal* language. Get in the habit of consciously changing these self-explanations using *temporary, specific,* and *external* terms, even if you don't really believe them in the beginning. Failure, when viewed through the correct lens, is merely delayed success. You should deal with your slips and falls as if they have no past and no future. If you try something and fail, then in your next attempt, you should forget about the previous failure. Failure is a common and temporary occurrence along the path to success. When things go badly, do not allow yourself to indulge in blind generalizations. Be specific and get to the heart of the matter. The more specific you can be in addressing that failure, the quicker you'll rebound from it. Finally, don't look for fixed personal character flaws to blame for your shortcomings. There is nothing useful in this search and it will steal your confidence to push on.

> ***F**ailure, when viewed through the correct lens, is merely delayed success.*

Your mental toughness depends on these inner explanations. Do not allow the old "tapes" to fill your head with nonsensical garbage like, "Here we go again," "You don't have what it takes," or "You always choke." Not only are these self-explanations inaccurate, but they are inconsistent with your dream and the commitment that you've made to pursue it.

As a coach, you're in a significant position to positively influence your athletes' inner explanations. Since most committed athletes respect their coaches, your words will occupy considerable "airtime" in their heads. Frequently athletes take the coach's word as the absolute truth. Your responsibility, then, is to be sure that you don't use *permanent, pervasive,* or *personal* language in explaining their failures to them. Telling a team after a loss that they're just a bunch of losers (permanent, pervasive, and personal) and have no talent (personal) won't do anything but further erode their confidence and eliminate what little mental toughness may be present on the squad. Those comments uttered in the heat of the moment do not motivate your players to work harder and do not provide them with anything constructive to work on.

If the value of failure is to be found in its learning experience, then before you speak, ask yourself, "What do I want my athletes to learn from this?" Asking yourself this question will frequently short-circuit permanent, pervasive, or personal comments that you might be tempted to make. Furthermore, it will save you from losing your athletes' respect and being labeled a bad coach.

For example, last year my daughter Sara returned from junior high softball practice angry and upset. As a new pitcher, she had been looking forward to that day's practice, because all the pitchers were going to get an opportunity to work with the high school varsity coach. Sara explained through tears that while the coach had made constructive suggestions to the two other pitchers, she hadn't said anything to her. When Sara finally got up the courage to ask the coach how she was doing and what she needed to work on, the woman turned to her and snapped, "Goldberg, you reek!!! You're doing everything wrong. You just reek!" Besides being inappropriate and completely useless, the coach's comments were personal and pervasive, leaving my daughter feeling terrible about herself *and* the coach.

When your athletes fail or succeed, be aware of *what* you say and *how* you say it. You can create mental toughness on a team by using the right language to explain setbacks and failures. Use permanent, pervasive, and personal language only to explain athletic successes. Otherwise, be specific in describing your athletes' failures, help them constructively externalize them, and explain them as temporary phenomena.

To help you more effectively guard against permanent, pervasive, and personal statements, fortify your defenses. Be internally alert and ready to pounce on these negative self-explanations whenever adversity strikes. Here's how.

The ABCs of Mental Toughness

A failure or setback (point A in figure 9.2) generates self-talk to explain this event (point B in figure 9.2). The self-talk can be either positive or negative. If it's positive, it is filled with language that is temporary, specific, and external (for example, "Today was too cold to play well," "I didn't get enough sleep last night," or "You guys were too nervous before the start; you need to learn a relaxation technique."). If your self-talk is negative, then your language is loaded with permanent, pervasive, and personal terms (such as, "I'm such a klutz," "The coach will never play me," or "I always manage to screw up when it counts."). Your self-explanations for the failure lead to point C in figure 9.2, or how you end up feeling. These emotions then have a significant impact on your mental toughness.

For example, positive self-talk in point B will lead to positive emotions in point C, emotions that reflect an underlying sense of hopefulness. To persevere in the face of adversity, you need these feelings of hopefulness. Furthermore, this hopefulness energizes you to experience other mental

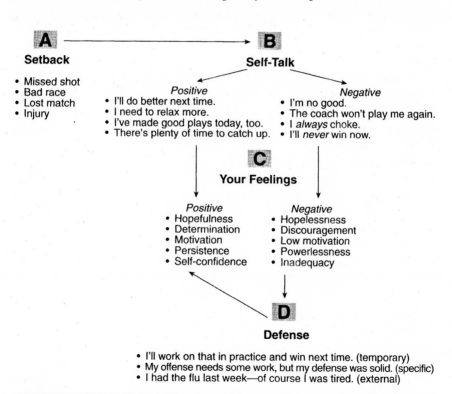

Figure 9.2 The ABCs of mental toughness.

toughness components, like determination, self-confidence, motivation, and persistence. A negative self-explanation in point B, on the other hand, will lead to an overall negative feeling in point C, a feeling of hopelessness. When you're feeling hopeless, mental toughness is virtually impossible to maintain. Hopelessness kills your physical and psychic energy, undermining your will. This leads to other failure-generating emotions like discouragement, inadequacy, powerlessness, and low motivation.

If your self-explanations for failure leave you feeling hopeless and defeated, then you need to add some defense, point D in the diagram. This defense involves interrupting the negative self-talk of point B and then countering it with language that is more positive, temporary, specific, and external in nature. This ABC formula is based on the work of Ellis and Harper, rational emotive therapists.[6] Their assumption was that your *thoughts* determine how you *feel*. Since your feelings, in turn, significantly impact your mental toughness and ability to persevere in the face of hardship, it is critical that you learn to change your thoughts (self-talk).

How do you employ this defense? Let's say, for example, that your automatic response to a failure is, "You're such a choke. You never come through when it counts. You don't even deserve to be on this team." If you let these negative self-explanations (point B) go on uninterrupted, you'll be left feeling worthless and inadequate, ready to pack it in at the next setback. Your defense might include countering statements like, "I made only one error all game, and that was when the ball took a bad hop. My offense was solid. The game wouldn't have gone to overtime if it wasn't for me. I did get too nervous on that last play, but I can correct that with practice. I don't always choke. In last week's game, I came through in the clutch. I'm one of the most solid players on this squad. Why else would I have been voted MVP last year?"

These counter-arguments involve positive statements that qualify the failure in more *specific*, *temporary*, and *external* ways. In addition, they also provide contradictory evidence to the seemingly factual nature of the negative evaluations. Getting in the habit of responding in this self-defensive way will leave you feeling more confident, motivated, and energized (point D in the diagram) to continue your quest. You can actively work on building up your mental-toughness muscles with regular practice of this ABCD sequence following a setback or failure.

Conclusion

As we've discussed, experiences of failure carry with them predictable emotions. Feeling embarrassed, inadequate, confused, saddened, discouraged, frustrated, and hopeless are all normal responses to striking out with the bases loaded, dropping the game-winning catch, blowing the game-saving free throws, or running the worst race of your life. While these emotions appear to indicate that all is lost, don't be deceived. The feelings of failure are in reality the doorway to ultimate success.

Most athletes feel uncomfortable when faced with these emotions and tend to move away from them. However, by avoiding situations where you might feel incompetent, embarrassed, or confused, you'll rob yourself of the opportunity to learn and grow as an athlete. Furthermore, experiences of failure make you mentally tougher and get you closer to your goals. Don't fear failure. It marks the doorway to your dreams. Train yourself to positively reframe your failures and setbacks. The feelings of failure let you know that you're taking risks and moving in the right direction. Get excited about your failures like home-run king Babe Ruth. The Babe was once asked how he felt after striking out. "I get excited," he responded, "because I know I'm one swing closer to a home run."

What would happen to your training and performances if you adopted this winning attitude? How could any slump or setback possibly affect you when you get more motivated after a failure? This reaction to setbacks is the heart of becoming mentally tough. If you get knocked down once, get up once. If you get knocked down twice, get up twice. If you get knocked down eight times, get up nine. The last time you get up, it will be to claim your prize.

In the last step of our model, you will learn how to build on your self-confidence and mental toughness to develop an "insurance policy" against future slumps. While poor performances can't be completely prevented, you can dramatically limit the impact that these occasional bad outings have on your game. When Step 10 is combined with the preceding steps' strategies, you can be assured that any performance difficulty you encounter will be short-lived.

As I've discussed in this step, your "reboundability" from failures is a key component of mental toughness. Step 10 will address a second critical component of mental toughness— your ability to stay calm and composed under competitive pressure. Both of these elements combine to provide a powerful one–two punch to knock out that slump and keep it down for the count.

STEP

10

INSURING AGAINST FUTURE SLUMPS

"The condition of your mind and body is a direct result of the conditioning of your mind and body."

—Dr. Rob Gilbert

The final step in the slump-busting model is to develop an "insurance policy" against future slumps. While no one can completely prevent bad performances, you can insure two things: (1) these subpar outings will be the exception, not the rule, in your athletic career; and (2) your failures and disappointments will not plant themselves in your front yard and blossom into long-term slumps. Remember, slumps need your cooperation to stay active and disruptive. You have to think in a set way, make specific nasty comments to yourself before and during performances, watch negative images before the start, and concentrate on all the wrong things in order for a slump to control you.

Like a parasite, a slump needs to be fed by *you*, the "host," to stay healthy. Ultimately *you* are the one with the power to starve that pesky performance-sucker into oblivion. Slump busting is about training your mind so that the *normal* ups and downs in sports have no *lasting* negative impact on your confidence or play. The overall purpose of the slump-busting model is not just to eliminate these repeated performance lows, but also to turn you into a mentally tough competitor. This mental toughness serves as a kind of insurance policy, helping you avoid future slumps.

In the previous step we discussed mental toughness as a psychic resilience or an ability to quickly rebound from setbacks and failures, fueled by a dogged persistence and refusal to quit until the goal has been achieved. A second critical element of mental toughness is the ability to stay calm, physically and mentally, before and during pressure-packed performances. This reboundability and "grace under fire" form an important part of your slump insurance. If your failures don't keep you down and you're able to handle the stress of competition effectively, then you will be less vulnerable to the conditions and situations that foster slumps.

> **I**f your failures don't keep you down and you're able to handle the stress of competition effectively, then you will be less vulnerable to the conditions and situations that foster slumps.

The main purpose of this final step in the slump-busting model is two-fold: (1) to help you recognize the early-warning signs of performance-disrupting stress before it can negatively affect your performance; and (2) to help you effectively and consistently control your level of physiological arousal, using the techniques presented in this and other steps in the model. Your ability to control your arousal level will contribute to your sense of confidence, control, and mental toughness.

Most athletes who struggle with repeated performance difficulties share a number of problems that directly contribute to their slumps. We've discussed several to this point, including poor concentration, fears, low self-confidence, negative thinking, performance-disrupting imagery, and a lack of belief in one's self. One of the *key* contributing problems, however, is an inability to stay cool in the clutch. Slumping athletes frequently get too nervous for their own good. Whether they are preoccupied with "not messing up again" or pressuring themselves with "got tos," their physical and mental tension ties their muscles in knots and makes peak performance impossible. Conditioning yourself to better handle competitive pressure will not only help you break that slump, but also will ensure that future performance problems will be fleeting.

Every athlete who has ever choked knows the devastating power of nervousness run amuck. Out-of-control nerves can vanquish even the most talented and well-conditioned athlete. Uncontrolled stress can keep you sleepless the night before the big competition, steal your confidence, and sap your energy. Runaway nerves can quickly turn your big dream into a nightmare by sending you out too fast at the race's start, tricking you into trying too hard, or distracting you from your defensive assignment.

Behind a champion's impassive exterior is an inner knowledge that no matter how hot the competition gets, he or she will always remain cool inside. A champion is the personification of the eye of a hurricane, that totally calm spot at the center of the storm. As we discussed in Steps 2 and 3, mental toughness and the ability to maintain composure is significantly affected by concentration. Understanding that performance-disrupting stress stems from concentrating on uncontrollables, mentally tough athletes focus only on the things they can control: *themselves* and *their reactions* to the uncontrollables.

Slumping athletes, on the other hand, are preoccupied with a whole host of uncontrollables, and this focus raises their anxiety so high that their muscles refuse to respond as trained. Instead of being able to constructively harness their pregame jitters, their nerves get the best of them. To avoid slumps, then, you must not only learn to control your focus of concentration, but also learn to master your nerves.

Figure 10.1 presents the theoretical relationship between stress (physiological arousal) and performance. The vertical axis measures quality of performance. Anything low on the vertical axis represents poor performance. Anything high on the vertical axis represents those times when you're in the zone. The horizontal axis measures levels of physiological arousal: anxiety, stress, or nervousness. If you are on the far left side of the horizontal axis, you aren't psyched up. If you're on the far right side of the horizontal axis, you're too psyched up, perhaps to the point of "freaking out."

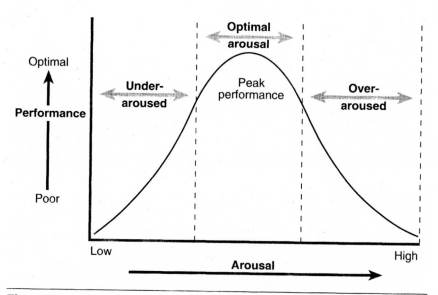

Figure 10.1 The relationship between stress and performance.

As the inverted-U shape of the graph line indicates, an athlete's performance begins to improve with increasing levels of arousal or excitement until it reaches a peak. At that point, further increases in stress cause a deterioration in the quality of the performance. Occasionally performance problems come from disinterest and under-arousal. When athletes go into a performance under-aroused, their performance will be flat and uninspired. Being overconfident is an example of under-arousal. Athletes or teams can get into trouble entering a competition overconfident. If the opponent begins to play exceedingly well, that under-arousal can quickly lead to panic (over-arousal), poor performance, and the big upset. Similarly, under-arousal from disinterest or not caring will lead to uninspired play. An athlete who doesn't want to compete puts forth a half-hearted effort with predictably subpar results.

Optimal arousal means that the athletes' level of physiological arousal is "just right" as they enter the competitive arena. They are "up" for the performance, and this excitement will maximize their chances of doing well. Athletes who enter the competitive arena looking forward to the challenge in this way will most often perform at their best. Over-arousal, on the other hand, means that the athletes are "over-amped" or too excited. Over-arousal frequently produces a sense of dread or foreboding as the athletes prepare to enter the competition. A physiological state of over-arousal is almost always present when athletes choke. Most athletes who struggle with slumps are experiencing too much anxiety just before their performance begins.

It's important to understand that the performance–arousal relationship varies widely among individual athletes. That is, every athlete responds to stress differently. Some athletes seem to tolerate high levels of stress comfortably, while others tend to get knocked off track by relatively low levels of nervousness. As a result, situations that psych up one athlete to peak performance may not be enough to get a second athlete out of an under-aroused state and may send a third athlete into over-arousal and poor performance. Coaches should be aware of these individual differences, so that they can better tailor what they say to their athletes and teams before and at breaks in the competition.

The effect of physiological arousal also depends on your sport and the specific athletic actions you perform within that sport. Sports that involve fine motor movement and delicate balancing of hand–eye coordination and timing are more susceptible to performance-disrupting stress than those involving more gross motor movement. Thus, the actions of returning a serve, shooting a foul shot, throwing a pitch, putting a 30 footer, or kicking a field goal are more vulnerable to disruption by increasing stress levels than are blocking in football, running cross-country, wrestling, or powerlifting.

Reading Preperformance Nervousness

Mentally tough athletes have two skills that set them apart from their slumping counterparts. First, they have the ability to consciously or unconsciously *read* the kind of preperformance nervousness they are experiencing. Second, they can change their level of physiological arousal as needed. For example, five minutes before tip-off, if these athletes recognize that they are getting too anxious, they can quickly calm themselves and get back up to optimal arousal. On the other hand, if they "read" that they are under-aroused, they can psych themselves up to optimal arousal.

In Step 2 I discussed the foundation for positive change in sports as *awareness*. You have to know what you're doing wrong physically or technically before you can correct it. The same holds true for handling competitive pressure. Before you can master it and consistently get to an optimal arousal level, you must have an awareness of what under- and over-arousal look and feel like. For example, if you miss the early-warning signs of excessive physiological arousal, you may not have time to do anything constructive about it once the performance begins. Your ability to stay cool in the clutch depends on how well you can learn to read your physiological signals.

> **Y**our ability to stay cool in the clutch depends on how well you can learn to read your physiological signals.

You read preperformance nervousness three ways:

1. In your body by how it *feels*
2. In your mind by how and what you *think*
3. In your behavior by how you *act*

The Feelings of Optimal and Over-Arousal

Since the vast majority of slumps are caused by over-arousal, our discussion will focus on that problem, though I will briefly touch on how to read under-arousal. In the following example, we will examine the feelings, thoughts, and actions of optimal and over-arousal.

Joyce was a professional triathlete who struggled with a slump that was primarily the result of too much prerace nervousness. Before her swimming leg, the first of the triathlon (swimming, cycling, and running), she would worry about falling too far behind, how weak a swimmer she was, how much bigger and better her opponents were, and past races in which she'd been unable to erase the deficit caused by a lousy swim. Her negative focus was a bigger liability than any real limitations in size, stroke technique, or stamina. Joyce's problem wasn't being a "bad swimmer." It was being over-aroused.

Since you can read over-arousal in your body by how it feels, how did Joyce experience over-arousal? Ten to fifteen minutes before the start of her subpar races, Joyce experienced a predictable set of feelings in her body. Her nervousness seemed to settle low in her stomach, leaving her feeling sick. Her arms and legs felt incredibly heavy. In addition, she felt completely exhausted, regardless of how much rest she had gotten the previous night. These body feelings almost always preceded a bad performance and constituted her *physical signs* of over-arousal. A year before this slump, Joyce had one satisfying triathlon that had started with a great swim. To achieve a peak performance, she must have been at the optimal arousal level before the start. What were these good feelings of nervousness? She had a sensation of "butterflies" high in her chest. Her arms and legs felt light and energized. She felt totally alert and pumped, as if she had unlimited strength and endurance. These body sensations she described constituted her *physical signs* of optimal arousal.

The Thoughts of Optimal and Over-Arousal

As described above, Joyce's prerace thoughts during her slump were mostly negative and pressure-inducing. She'd compare herself with all the other athletes, remember past bad swims, question whether she had trained hard enough, and threaten herself with imagined negative consequences if she failed again (like, "You've got to do better this race. You're going to lose your sponsorship money unless you place in the top five. You've got to prove yourself to them."). Predictably, these kinds of thoughts always preceded her bad swims. This self-talk represented the *mental signs* of Joyce's over-arousal. In last year's only great triathlon, her prerace thoughts were completely different and had little to do with her race (such as, "There's absolutely no pressure today because this race doesn't even matter. This will be fun. I haven't seen Sammi, Jen, or Alice in so long. I can't wait until tonight to be able to catch up with what they've been doing. What a great day today."). These thoughts represented her *mental signs* of optimal arousal.

The Actions of Optimal and Over-Arousal

Every athlete *acts* differently just before the big competition. Joyce's bad races were almost always preceded by the following ritual: After her warm-ups, she would sit quietly by herself and watch the other racers. Then she would cover her head with a towel and try to block them out by mentally rehearsing the swimming leg over and over again. These were Joyce's *behavioral signs* of over-arousal. Before last year's good race, Joyce did not sit at all. Instead, she bounced around, chatting with her husband, talking and joking with close friends, and moving constantly. These prerace actions constituted her *behavioral signs* of optimal arousal.

Dwayne was a high school basketball standout who was referred to me by his coach halfway through his junior season. An all-conference player, team captain, and top scorer, Dwayne was suddenly having problems with his "nerves" before all his games. On game day he felt lethargic and exhausted, regardless of how much sleep he had gotten the night before. As game time approached he started to feel sick to his stomach, and just before the team went out on the floor he'd invariably vomit.

What was especially puzzling for everyone involved was that Dwayne had never experienced any of this as a starting player during his freshman and sophomore years. He was always calm before his games and started them with confidence and intensity. All of this suddenly changed as he entered his junior year. For the first 10 games of the season the coach had to bench him early because Dwayne could barely get up and down the court. Although he'd settle down and regain his strength by halftime, he was of no use to the team the entire first half. His parents called me after a physical examination ruled out any medical problems.

Dwayne's problem seemed to start the summer before his junior year. Because his sophomore year had been so successful, he began to attract the attention of colleges all over the country. That summer he had been invited to attend a prestigious blue-chip basketball camp, a dream come true. With college scouts coming out of the woodwork, Dwayne began to think too much about how they would view him. Would he be good enough? Would he get a full scholarship? Could he make it in Division I? Rather than approaching game day the way he had in the past, with excitement and enthusiasm, Dwayne now felt burdened, wondering how many scouts would be in the stands and whether he'd play well enough to impress them. His worries brewed all day so that by game time he was exhausted and nauseated. Vomiting made him even more anxious and further contributed to his performance difficulties.

Dwayne was clearly in a state of over-arousal before his games. By learning to get control of his runaway nerves, he would be able to

→

conserve his energy, keep his lunch down, and play up to his potential. The first step was to help him see how focusing on uncontrollables like the reactions of college scouts, getting a scholarship, what others would think about him, his future in basketball, and so on was contributing to his nervousness. Instead Dwayne learned to keep his game day and pregame focus on himself and things that he could control.

Next, I taught Dwayne the resource-room exercise (shown in this chapter) and how to do slow, diaphragmatic breathing. Dwayne went to his resource room every night before bed and soon began to go there on game day and just before the tip-off. During timeouts and when necessary, he used the deep breathing to stay calm and centered. After two weeks of daily practice, Dwayne's exhaustion and pregame vomiting disappeared. Just as quickly, his pregame energy level returned and he was able to start games with the same kind of intensity and composure that he had shown the previous two years.

It soon became clear to Joyce that she *felt*, *thought*, and *acted* differently before her good and bad races. Recognizing these personal signs of optimal and over-arousal enabled her to begin to develop a strategy for controlling her level of physiological arousal. This awareness forms your first line of defense in managing stress. For example, Joyce changed her prerace ritual so that she no longer sat by herself, analyzing and mentally rehearsing the race. She stopped her strategy and planning sessions two nights before the competition. She realized that she was the kind of athlete who did better by completely blocking the race out of her mind before the start of the competition. Whenever she felt heavy and exhausted and had a strong urge to sit alone with her race thoughts (her feelings, behaviors, and thoughts that signal over-arousal), she forced herself instead to physically jump around and distract herself in nonrace conversation (her behaviors and thoughts that accompany optimal arousal).

The Feelings, Thoughts, and Actions of Under-Arousal

Let's say that you are the exception to the rule and you can link your performance troubles directly to a state of under-arousal. What kind of body feelings, thoughts, and behaviors might be present? The main physiological signs of under-arousal are lethargy and fatigue. In addition, you may experience feelings of heaviness in your arms and legs. Evidence of under-arousal may also be thoughts totally unrelated to performance (for example, "Should I go to the prom with Bill or Alex?" or "I wonder what courses I should take next year."), thoughts that reflect a state of overconfidence (such as, "She's terrible; this will be a piece of cake!" or "They don't have a chance against us. . . I wonder who we'll play in the next round."), or self-talk that genuinely reflects disinterest (such as, "Why am I even here? I couldn't care less about this match. . . This is so stupid."). The behaviors of under-arousal are in keeping with the sense of physical lethargy and fatigue (lying around, sitting quietly, or sleeping) or reflect a state of overconfidence (joking around or poking fun at the opponents).

EVALUATING YOUR PREPERFORMANCE AROUSAL

An important part of your slump insurance entails learning how to accurately read your level of preperformance nervousness. Like many of the skills discussed in this book, mastery takes practice. To improve your "reading skills," closely examine two or more of your good and bad performances (those that clearly represent your slump or block) in the following way:

1. Starting with your first bad performance, put an "x" on figure 10.1 where you think you were on the curve just before the action began. How under- or over-aroused were you?

2. As you think back to this performance, record on a piece of paper in as much detail as possible what you remember *feeling* in your body (the physical signs of arousal), the kinds of *thinking* you engaged in (the mental signs of arousal), and how you *acted* before the start (the behavioral signs of arousal).

3. Repeat #1 and #2 for one or two other bad performances to familiarize yourself with your signs of under- or over-arousal.

4. Follow #1 through #3 for two or more good performances to discover your signs of optimal arousal.

You may not notice a clear-cut difference among under-, optimal, and over-arousal in all three areas like Joyce did. However, by carefully examining enough performances, you will discover the one or two crucial differences that you can then use as early-warning indicators for you to take action and move yourself back up the curve to optimal arousal.

Lowering Over-Arousal

Through the course of this book, we've discussed a number of ways that you can cool yourself down when the heat of competition has been turned up. Switching your focus of concentration (Steps 2 and 3), changing or stopping negative self-talk (Step 5), using coping and mastery imagery (Step 6), and using the relaxation scripts from these imagery exercises all will help you constructively channel your nervousness into peak performance.

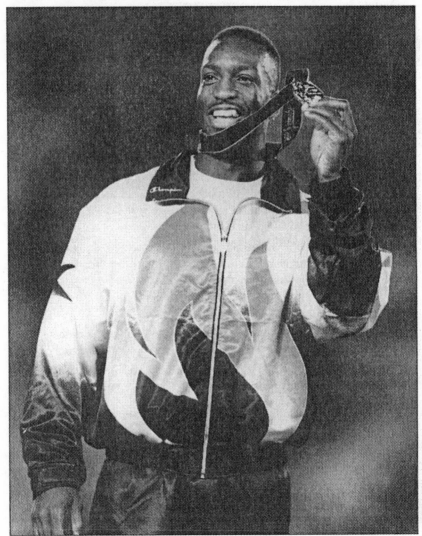

© Associated Sports Photography/George Herringshaw

Other helpful techniques are progressive muscle relaxation, autogenic training, and breath control training. (See the appendix for detailed instructions.) You can use any of these techniques to calm yourself down before performance and return yourself to an optimal level of arousal. These three relaxation techniques can also be used before your imagery sessions in place of the ones we discussed in Step 6.

Here is one additional cooling down strategy that I've found valuable for developing mental toughness and helping slumping athletes master the pressure of competition. This technique makes use of imagery and the phenomenon of dissociation (mentally separating yourself from your surroundings) to create a special "resource room" where athletes can go before the performance to help them remain calm, confident, and focused. As an arousal control tool, the resource room will help you tame the disruptive nervousness so common in a slump.

The resource room is a powerful arousal-control tool that can help you better handle the heat of competition and ward off slumps. The secret to its effectiveness is simple: *practice*. If you spend enough "time" in your resource room, it will become readily available to you when you need it. Spending 5 to 10 minutes there nightly before sleep may be an optimal time for you to fine-tune this safe haven.

You need not practice both the resource room and your imagery exercises on the same night. While some athletes go to their resource room first and then practice mental rehearsal from there, you may not want to do this. In fact, combining these exercises may be too distracting for you. Instead, you may find it easier to set aside separate nights for imagery and resource-room practice. With consistent practice, you'll also begin to notice that your "energy" or "confidence" machines begin to really work. One high school swimmer whose energy machine was a waterfall claimed that, in the middle of her longer races, she drew strength from spontaneously hearing the waterfall's roar as she swam.

CREATING AND USING YOUR RESOURCE ROOM

■ Your Safe Haven

Briefly think about a safe place where you can go in your mind's eye and feel completely removed, relaxed, comfortable, and confident. Your resource room can be a real place, a product of your imagination, or some combination of these. It can be outdoors, indoors, or both. It can be a spot where you've been before or somewhere "over

→

the rainbow" that you've never visited. Let your imagination be your guide as you begin this exercise. Finally, you may want to make your own audiotape recording of the instructions for maximum benefit. If you decide to do this, remember to pause for 2 to 3 seconds when you see the series of dots (. . .).

■ Preliminary Relaxation

Sitting or lying comfortably in an environment free from distraction, gently close your eyes and focus your attention entirely on your breathing. . . . Keeping your rate and depth of respiration as normal as possible, simply notice the air coming in and going out from your nose or mouth. . . . If you prefer, focus on your breathing by feeling the rise and fall of your lower belly. . . . Every time your mind begins to wander, gently bring your attention back to this focus on your breathing. . . . Spend one or two minutes noticing your breath in this way until you become aware of yourself beginning to slow down and relax. . . .

■ The Stairs

As you sit or lie there comfortably, imagine yourself standing in front of a set of stairs. . . . The stairs may go up or down. . . . They may be made of wood, stone, grass, sand, or something else. . . . They may split or spiral as they go up or down. . . . And as you look at these stairs, notice that on a number of them are special containers with covers. These containers may look like hand-carved wooden boxes, ornate jars with lids, metal lock boxes, or special capsules. . . .And as you move to the first step . . . you go over to the container, open it, and remove something that you'd find quite useful as an athlete. . . . Perhaps you take out courage . . . or persistence . . . or calmness . . . and before you move to the next stair, think of something that you'd like to be rid of . . . something that's been a burden to you lately . . . that you can put into the container and seal away forever. . . . You may put in self-doubts . . . or a past bad performance . . . and once you've closed the lid, move to the next stair. . . . As you do, you notice that you begin to feel lighter and more relaxed. . . . And as you continue to move along that staircase, stop at the next container and remove something else you'd like to have . . . perhaps a championship focus . . . mental toughness . . . a positive attitude . . . And then put in that container something else that you'd like to let go of. In this container, for example, you might put negativity . . . a disturbing comment from another athlete or coach . . . or even an opponent or individual who is annoying you. . . . And after you do this, seal the lid and continue along the stairway. . . . At your own comfortable pace, move all the way up or down to the end . . . stopping as desired to pick up what you need and get rid of what you don't . . . until you find yourself at the end of those stairs.

■ Creating a Resource Room

From this place at the end of the stairs, imagine that you can travel to or are already at your resource room. . . . Whether your journey takes time or is instantaneous, find a way to enter that special place. . . . You may walk down a corridor to get there . . . or hop on the back of a bird or dolphin. . . . Let your imagination find the best way to move to that safe place in your mind where you can feel secure and protected. . . . It really doesn't matter how you get there. . . . You begin to look around. . . . What is it about this environment that makes it such a safe and special place? . . . Are there familiar sights that let you know you're protected and far away? . . . Are there colors that catch your eye? . . . or familiar movements? . . . If you are at a beach, for example, you can see the rhythmic movement of the waves as they break on the shore and then recede. . . . You may even notice the light sparkling and dancing off the water as it moves. . . . Every resource room has a special look that you can explore now. . . . And as you do that, what can you add to that safe place that will increase your comfort and confidence? . . . Will you hang evidence of your successes and triumphs around you? . . . trophies, medals, ribbons? . . . comments from your supporters? . . . Will your resource room have special pictures or posters that remind you of your dream and help you stay on track? . . . Maybe someone you really trust is in that room with you . . . or maybe you're alone or supported by a special friend or coach. . . . You can choose who and what will surround you to keep you confident and in control. . . .

Every resource room has familiar sounds that you can hear now. . . . Whether you hear the sound of water moving . . . the wind blowing . . . special music . . . or something entirely different isn't important. . . . You may hear the comforting sounds of your own breathing or the sounds of silence. . . . And every resource room has sensations that you become aware of now. . . . If you're outdoors, you may feel a breeze caressing your face . . . the air temperature against your skin. . . maybe the warmth of the sun . . . or something else. . . . And

→

if you're in that special room indoors, you may be surprised at the sensations you can feel now. . . . And as you become more aware of these sensations, you can feel more secure and more protected. . . . Every resource room provides the privacy you need to feel more and more confident. . . . This space is open only to you . . . and you alone decide who or what you'll allow to enter. . . '.

And as you feel more comfortable in this space, look around that room and find your "energy machine." . . . Think about an experience of suddenly getting a second wind . . . of feeling the fatigue melt away . . . and in its place you feel a renewed energy and determination. . . . Your energy machine could look like an old-fashioned coiled radiator . . . or something out of Star Trek with flashing lights and beeping computer boards . . . or it could be a rushing river, waves, or a waterfall. . . . It could simply be the warmth of the sun or a fire. . . . Your energy machine could look like a CD player that plays an energizing song. . . . There are no limits on what your energy machine looks like or how it operates. . . . Perhaps you'd like to try it out right now . . . hooking yourself up to it . . . turning it on. . . . Feel the energy beginning to move into you or simply see it happening . . . or maybe you're more aware of hearing the energy begin to move. . . . It really doesn't matter if you feel the energy flow into you . . . or see it flow into you . . . or only hear its movements. . . . In fact, your experience of the energy machine may be entirely different than this. . . . You can create your energy machine any way that works for you. . . .

You may simply make the energy machine a "confidence dispenser" . . . and when you "hook yourself up," you experience the confidence growing inside of you. . . . Or you may use this concept to calm yourself down . . . turning on the flow of ice water so you can be cool in the clutch. . . .

So while you explore this special room and add those things that make you feel competent . . . you may even create a place where you practice your mental rehearsal . . . perhaps a special chair and screen where you can preview and review your great performances. . . . Take a few moments right now to memorize all the sights . . . sounds . . . and feelings of your resource room. . . . Perhaps take notes on the things you want to add when you come back here again. . . . You can add or subtract anything that you'd like in this place until it feels just right for you. . . .

And before you allow yourself to leave for now, memorize the feelings in your body right now. . . . What do your arms and legs feel like? . . . Are you aware of lightness or heaviness in your body? . . . What does your relaxation feel like? . . . When you next return to your resource room, these feelings will serve as your guide to help you get back to this place. . . . And after you've surveyed the relaxation in your body, slowly allow yourself to return to a normal waking state.

Raising Under-Arousal

While certainly less common, under-arousal can still be a slump-feeding problem for some athletes. If you struggle with not being psyched up enough before your performances, what can you do to constructively raise your nervousness to an optimal level? Try the following strategies:

• **Physically Raise Your Arousal Level**—Stand up, move, or bounce around; physically warm up harder or longer than usual to get your heart rate, respiration, and blood pressure up.

• **Deliberately Change Your Breathing**—Speed up your breathing and make it more shallow, deliberately breathing from your upper chest. Under-arousal is marked by very slow, diaphragmatic breathing. Change the rate and depth of your breathing, and you can increase your level of physiological arousal.

• **Change Your Self-Talk**—Under-arousal is usually accompanied by uninspired, disinterested self-talk. Deliberately change the dialogue of your inner coach so that he or she increases the importance of the contest and begins to pressure you.

• **Change Your Goals for the Performance**—If the outcome of the performance does not inspire you because your opponents are much less skilled than you are, you need to set more challenging, performance-related, process goals (see Step 7). These new goals can pertain to executing your offense or defense in a certain way, practicing a weaker part of your game, or playing a less-comfortable position.

• **Link the Present Performance to Your Big-Enough Why**—By making a conscious connection between today's performance and your ultimate athletic dream, you can sometimes generate more performance-enhancing stress. You can tell yourself that today is a dress rehearsal for that big contest, or you can use today to mentally practice competing against those tough opponents you're likely to face later.

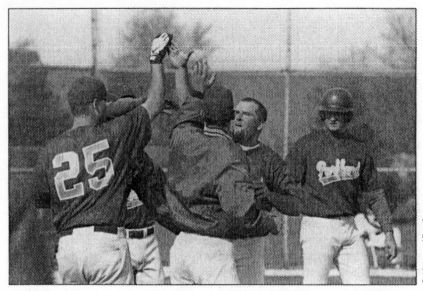

© Human Kinetics

The Slump Meter

The foundation of the slump-busting model and mental toughness in general lies in your awareness. Establishing self-control and building self-confidence is based on an *awareness* of the self-talk of your inner coach. Handling stress is based on an *awareness* of the focus of your concentration. Controlling your level of physiological arousal before competing depends on your ability to read yourself and an *awareness* of your anxiety level. Similarly, the best slump insurance you can possibly have is an *awareness* of the early-warning signs of an impending slump. If you know a slump's early-warning signs, then you can immediately take action to defuse it.

> ***T****he best slump insurance you can have is an awareness of the early-warning signs of an impending slump.*

How can you tell if a slump may be heading your way? Is there a measurable change in the atmospheric or barometric pressure? Does the relative humidity go up or down? Can you register it on a temperature or wind gauge? While these kinds of instruments won't pick up the sign of an impending slump, our handy slump meter will (see figure 10.2). The slump meter is based on a series of general questions that you should ask yourself periodically before and after a performance to let you know if the foul weather of a slump may be settling in your area.

THE SLUMP METER

■ Questionnaire

Answer True or False to each statement below.

1. The harder I try, the worse I get these days.
2. My self-talk before this performance was negative.
3. I was dreading the performance.
4. My concentration *during* the performance was in the past or the future.
5. I couldn't get over how strong, fast, big, or talented my opponents were before the start.
6. I kept seeing internal images of what I was afraid would occur.
7. Before I started, I was upset by something that had happened earlier.
8. My self-talk has a lot of "Here we go again," "This always happens," and "I never" in it.
9. I found myself evaluating and criticizing my performance while it was going on.
10. I worried about failing before or during the performance.
11. I was singing the what-ifs before or during the performance.
12. I feel incredibly frustrated with my performances lately.
13. I focus on mechanics and instruct myself a great deal, especially during a performance.
14. I was not having fun before or during the performance.
15. I found myself carrying my mistakes around with me the entire time.
16. I kept remembering past examples of lousy performances.
17. I'm having trouble remembering the last time I had a decent performance.
18. I noticed that I've been trying too hard lately.
19. Even though everyone says my problem is mental, I'm still convinced it's my mechanics.
20. I find myself thinking too much throughout the performance.

■ Reading the Slump Meter

Each statement above represents a potential mental mistake that a slumping athlete can make. If you're beginning to regularly commit too many

→

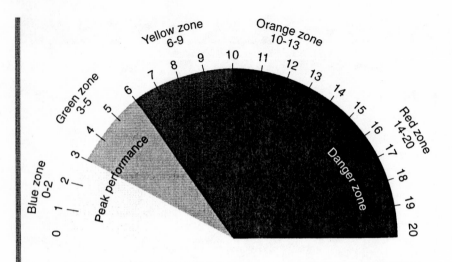

Figure 10.2 The slump meter.

of these kinds of mental errors, then you may be headed for a slump. Start at zero on the slump meter in figure 10.2. For each statement above that you marked True, move yourself one space up the meter. The slump meter has been divided into five zones: Blue, Green, Yellow, Orange, and Red. In that order, each zone represents an increasing susceptibility to a slump or block. Scores in the Blue Zone (0 to 2) mean that your mental state is right for peak performance. Scores in the Green Zone (3 to 5), while not reflective of the same degree of mental toughness as the Blue Zone, indicate that you're holding your own and not in any immediate danger of slumping. Scores in the Yellow (6 to 9), Orange (10 to 13), and Red (14 to 20) zones reflect increasing amounts of dangerous slump thinking that will likely cause a performance crash. To determine what zone you're in, simply add up the number of True answers and find the corresponding zone that includes that number. For example, a total of three puts you in the Green Zone, while a total of 15 puts you in the Red Zone. If your scores on the slump meter begin to leave the Green Zone at any time, then you need to quickly review and begin to use the slump-busting strategies in this book.

Conclusion

The 10-step model presented in this book will help you persevere. It provides an antidote to a slump as well as the skills to help you ward off future performance problems. Working with the strategies described in each step will help you develop the mental toughness that will serve as your slump insurance. While no one is completely immune to bad performances, you can train yourself to shorten those that do come your way.

Endurance-sport athletes train their bodies hard in order to withstand the rigors of their contests. Without the proper conditioning, physical fitness is impossible to maintain, and these athletes will fade at some point in their competition. Their high level of strength and endurance serves a preventative role, making them less vulnerable under stress to a physical breakdown.

Similarly, without the proper mental conditioning, the athlete becomes more susceptible to bouts with slumps. A high level of mental fitness helps the athlete master the pressure of competition and effectively ward off slumps. As a serious athlete, you would never leave your physical training and conditioning to chance. Why leave your slump-busting mental fitness to chance? Lucky socks or that favorite Barney underwear will never be as confidence-inspiring or as reliable as the feeling of mental toughness born of systematic practice of these techniques.

You can take active control and bust slumps by

- Step 1: Ruling out their nonmental causes
- Step 2: Developing an awareness of the role that you play in feeding the slump and reestablishing self-control
- Step 3: Keeping yourself focused on what's important and blocking everything else out
- Step 4: Taking action to defeat your fears
- Step 5: Learning to expect success and believe in yourself
- Step 6: Developing the ability to mentally see what you want to happen before it does
- Step 7: Setting slump-busting goals and creating a big-enough why to help you persevere
- Step 8: Building self-confidence
- Step 9: Bolstering your mental toughness by developing the ability to quickly rebound from setbacks and adversity
- Step 10: Developing a good slump-insurance policy to effectively handle future performance lows

After you've toughened yourself in these ways, you can still wear that lucky underwear for an extra edge!

A P P E N D I X
RELAXATION EXERCISES

Progressive Muscle Relaxation[1]

Relaxation is a crucial athletic skill that helps you

- handle the pressure of competition,
- physiologically cool down the body in between and after athletic events,
- maintain appropriate concentration, and
- prepare to visualize and mentally rehearse.

Preparation

Lie comfortably on your back, feet spread 18 inches apart, hands by your sides, palms up. Allow 20 minutes for this exercise in an environment free from distractions. You will be working your way through the muscle groups in your body, alternating contraction (tension) with relaxation. Contraction for 10 seconds should be to no more than 90 percent tightness. Remember to maintain relaxation in all other muscles except for those being used.

Note: If you're administering this exercise to a group of athletes, read the script slowly in a quiet tone of voice. The series of dots (. . .) indicates a 2 to 3 second pause. If you're using the script by yourself, making your own audiotape recording will make following the instructions without distractions much easier.

---

[1] This exercise is adapted from a workshop recording by Kenneth Ravizza (1984), University of Virginia.

Procedure

1. Begin to tighten all the muscles up and down your right leg until you reach 90 percent tension. (Pointing your toes either toward or away from your head, or raising your leg half an inch off the floor will help you increase the tension.) Hold this tension for 10 seconds. . . . Study the tension . . . feel it . . . and then repeat to yourself "let go," and as you do, slowly allow your leg to relax. Feel the tension flowing out your leg onto the surface that you're lying on. . . . Feel the difference in your leg now. . . . Inhale slowly, expanding your lower belly . . . pause, and then exhale. . . .

2. Repeat the procedure in #1 again for your right leg, paying close attention to the difference between being tight and loose. . . . Inhale and exhale slowly. . . .

3. Tighten all the muscles up and down your left leg, holding this tension for 10 seconds. . . . Notice these feelings of muscle tightness as you do so. . . . Hold it . . . and then repeat to yourself the words "let go," and as you hear the words, let all the tension in your left leg slowly drain out. . . . Note the sensations that accompany relaxation. . . . Do you feel a heaviness? . . . lightness? . . . warmth? . . . tingling? . . . or other feelings associated with looseness? . . . Inhale comfortably and slowly . . . and then exhale. . . .

4. Repeat the procedure for your left leg again . . . inhaling and exhaling comfortably at the end.

5. Tighten your buttocks muscles to 90 percent of your strength, holding the tension. . . . Remember to keep all the other muscles in your body relaxed. . . . Become aware of the feelings of tightness. . . . Hold this for 10 seconds and then repeat to yourself "let go" and as you do, let the tension flow out of this area. . . . Notice the change in sensations as the relaxation begins to replace the tightness. . . . Feel the looseness and inhale slowly and deeply . . . pause . . . and then exhale comfortably.

6. Repeat #5 for your buttocks muscles, followed by slow, deep breathing. . . .

7. Tighten your stomach or abdominal muscles and focus your attention on the sensations of tightness. . . . Hold the tension for 10 seconds while everything else in your body remains loose. . . . Hold the tension here . . . and then repeat to yourself "let go" . . . allowing your stomach muscles to soften and relax. . . . Study the difference as you feel the looseness here. . . . Inhale slowly and comfortably . . . pause . . . and then exhale. . . . Let the relaxation flow throughout your body. . . .

8. Repeat #7 once again, following the relaxation with one or two slow, deep, comfortable breaths. . . .

9. Tighten all the muscles in your chest and across the back of your shoulders (push your shoulder blades back and together). . . . As you hold the tension, study it. . . . Feel what tension in this part of your body feels like. . . . After 10 seconds, repeat "let go," and slowly let your shoulders and chest relax. . . . Feel the looseness, warmth, lightness, or other sensations of relaxation spreading into these muscles. . . . Inhale comfortably . . . pause . . . exhale slowly. . . .

10. Repeat #9 for your chest and shoulders. . . . Breathe slowly and comfortably . . . in and out. . . .

11. Tighten the muscles in both of your arms, slowly bringing the tension to 90 percent. Making fists will help you feel the tension up and down your arms. Notice the tension in all the muscles of your arms and hands. . . . Hold it and then "let go," allowing the tension to slowly flow out of your arms, down from your shoulders . . . through your upper arms, down through your lower arms . . . and out your hands and fingers. . . . Feel the relaxation replacing the tightness. . . . Study it. . . . Feel it. . . . Breathe in comfortably and deeply . . . and then breathe out. . . .

12. Repeat #11, studying the tension and relaxation. . . . Breathe in and out comfortably.

13. Tense the muscles in your neck by pressing down with your head into the surface where you are lying. Notice the tightness in this area. . . . Feel it for 10 seconds . . . then "let go," and allow the tension to drain out completely. Let the your neck muscles go limp and allow the underlying surface to completely support your head. . . . Inhale comfortably . . . pause . . . and exhale. . . .

14. Repeat #13, remembering to keep all the other muscles in your body loose. . . .

15. Tighten the muscles in your jaw by clenching your teeth. Feel the tension in this area. . . . Hold it for 10 seconds and then repeat those words to yourself "let go." . . . Slowly let your jaw muscles relax. . . . Let your lips relax and mouth begin to open slightly. . . . Feel the difference in this area. . . . Inhale and feel the relaxation . . . pause and then exhale slowly. . . .

16. Repeat #15, followed by slow, deep breathing. . . .

17. Tighten the muscles in your entire face, including your jaws. Grimace, furrow your brow, clench your teeth, and hold this tension. . . . Hold it. . . . Feel it, and then "let go" . . . letting all the tension drain from your face. Let your forehead and cheek muscles soften. . . . Let your jaw muscles relax again. . . . Feel the difference as you inhale comfortably . . . and then exhale.

18. Repeat the process for your face again. . . .

19. Now tighten all the muscles in your body to 90 percent tension. . . . Tighten your legs, arms, buttocks, abdomen, chest, shoulders, neck, jaws, and face. . . . Hold the tension and focus on it. . . . Then repeat those two words to yourself "let go," and slowly allow all the tension to drain away from your body. . . . Imagine all the tension being replaced by feelings of relaxation. . . . Study the difference. . . . Breathe in slowly . . . pause and then exhale. . . .

20. One final time tighten your entire body to 90 percent of your strength. . . . Hold the tension and then "let go." . . . Notice the feelings of relaxation as they spread around your body, flowing into every muscle. . . . If any areas remain tight in your body, tighten those muscles once more, holding the tension and then letting them relax. . . .

How to Practice

Like any athletic skill, relaxation is learned with proper and sufficient practice. Once daily at bedtime or when you first get up in the morning are times that usually work best. After two weeks of daily practice, it will be much easier for you to quickly recognize where you're holding your muscle tension and to "let it go." Soon you'll be able to do progressive muscle relaxation without needing to contract your muscles ahead of time. When skilled at this exercise, you'll only need to focus on your tension and use the mental command "let go" to get relaxed.

Autogenic Training[2]

Introduction

There are certain physiological sensations that regularly accompany the relaxation response: heaviness in the arms and legs; a feeling of warmth in the arms and legs; slower heart rate; slower, more even respiration; and a coolness in the forehead. Because your thoughts have a tremendous influence over your body, it is possible for you to control your level of relaxation by what you say to yourself. By repeatedly giving yourself the following suggestions in succession, you can achieve a relaxed state.

1. Feelings of heaviness in the arms and legs
2. Feelings of warmth in the arms and legs

---

[2] This exercise is based on the work of H. Benson (1975).

3. Cardiac control and regulation

4. Control over your respiration

5. Cooler forehead

Preparation

Sit comfortably in an environment free from distractions. Allow 20 minutes for the exercise. Read over the instructions before you begin, so that the sequence of suggestions will be clear in your mind. Close your eyes and develop a passive, let-it-happen attitude. Initially you may not be able to achieve all of the desired feelings. This is quite natural. Relax and keep practicing—soon you'll begin to experience all the feelings.

Note: If you're administering this exercise to a group of athletes, read the script slowly in a quiet tone of voice. The series of dots (. . .) indicates a 2 to 3 second pause. If you're using the script by yourself, making your own audiotape recording will make following the instructions without distractions much easier.

Procedure

1. Heaviness of the limbs. Repeat the following suggestions over and over again for about 4 minutes: "My hands are beginning to feel very heavy. . . . They are feeling heavier and heavier. . . . My arms are feeling heavier and heavier. . . . My legs are feeling heavier and heavier. . . . I can feel the heaviness moving up and down my hands, arms, and legs . . . heavier and heavier."

2. Warmth in the limbs. Repeat the following to yourself for 4 minutes: "My hands are beginning to feel warm. . . . They are feeling warmer and warmer. . . . The warmth is spreading up my arms . . . warmer and warmer. . . . My legs and feet are feeling warmer and warmer. . . . "

3. Cardiac regulation. Repeat the following for 4 minutes: "My heart is becoming slower and more regular. . . . It is beating slower and slower . . . slower and more consistent. . . . My heart rate is slowing down more and more . . . slower and slower. . . ."

4. Breathing regulation. Repeat the following to yourself for 4 minutes: "My breathing is becoming slower and more regular . . . slower and slower. . . . My breathing is very deep, slow, and regular . . . easy, slow, and regular."

5. Coolness in the forehead. Repeat for the 4-minute time period: "My forehead is beginning to feel cool. . . . It is feeling cooler and cooler . . . cooler and cooler."

Breath Control Training[3]

Preparation

Find a comfortable place to sit where you'll be free from distractions. Focus on your breathing throughout this exercise. Should you get distracted, quickly and gently bring yourself back to this target focus. Allow 5 minutes per practice session.

Procedure

1. Inhale deeply through your nostrils to a slow count of four, making sure that your diaphragm is expanding as you inhale. (You can keep one hand on your diaphragm or lower belly area and feel it rise as you inhale.) The process should be easy and relaxed, without strain. Your stomach and lower abdomen should be pushed out when you're finished with this inhalation.

2. Pause briefly.

3. Exhale through your mouth in a very slow and relaxed manner. As you do, slowly count to 10. You may hear an ahhhhhhh sound as you exhale like this. Your exhalation and counting should be effortless and easy. Feel your belly and diaphragm relax as you exhale. Shorten the count if necessary to keep your exhalation unforced.

4. Repeat #1 through #3 over and over again for the 5-minute practice period.

---

[3]This exercise is adapted from James Loehr, *Athletic Excellence* (1982).

NOTES

Step 1

1. Jenkins, 57.
2. Price, 36.

Step 3

1. For more information, see Ravizza and Hanson.

Step 4

1. Borges, "Hurst Is Down and Out as Patriot," 58.
2. Ibid.
3. Bandler, 37-48.

Step 5

1. Telander, 110.
2. Layden, "Now for the Hard Part," 62-65.

Step 7

1. Ferguson, 6-27.

Step 8

1. Ferguson, 4-17.
2. Ibid., 4-18.
3. Dorrance and Nash, 28.
4. Ibid., 34.

5. Reilly, "Goodness Gracious, He's a Great Ball of Fire," 66.
6. Ibid., 70.
7. Reilly, "Strokes of Genius," 35-49.

Step 9

1. Wolff, 156.
2. Seligman, 44.
3. Layden, "The Long Road Back," 44-50.
4. Taylor, 96.
5. Schumacher, D-1.
6. Ellis and Harper, 25.

BIBLIOGRAPHY

Bandler, R. 1985. *Using Your Brain for a Change*. Moab, UT: Real People Press.

Benson, H. 1975. *The Relaxation Response*. New York: William Morrow.

Borges, R. 1995. Hurst is down and out as Patriot—Parcells waives oft-beaten cornerback. *The Boston Globe*, 21 November, 57-59.

————. 1995. Agent says client has been playing hurt. *The Boston Globe*, 21 November, 57-59.

————, and J. Burris. 1995. Parcells fires back at agent—coach says Hurst never spoke of disc, nerve injuries. *The Boston Globe*, 23 November, 97, 102.

Callahan, G. 1996. Gasp. *Sports Illustrated*. Olympic Preview. 21 July, 98-101.

Canfield, J., and M.V. Hansen. 1993. *Chicken Soup for the Soul*. Deerfield Beach, FL: Health Communications.

Daggett, T., and J. Stone. 1992. *Dare to Dream*. Tarrytown, NY: Wynwood Press.

Demak, R. 1991. Mysterious malady. *Sports Illustrated*. 8 April, 44-49.

Dorrance, A., and T. Nash. 1996. *Training Soccer Champions*. Raleigh, NC: JTC Sports Inc.

Ellis, A., and R. Harper. 1975. *A New Guide to Rational Living*. North Hollywood, CA: Wilshire Books.

Ferguson, H.E. 1983. *The Edge*. Cleveland, OH: Getting the Edge.

Garfield, C., and H.Z. Bennett. 1984. *Peak Performance*. Los Angeles, CA: Jeremy P. Tarcher.

Gilbert, R. 1988. *Gilbert on Greatness*. Bloomfield, NJ: The Center for Sport Success.

Jackson, P., and H. Delehanty. 1995. *Sacred Hoops*. New York, NY: Hyperion.

Jenkins, S. 1995. Love and love. *Sports Illustrated*. 8 March, 52-61.

Kurkjian, T. 1996. Inside baseball: Young and gifted. *Sports Illustrated*. 1 July, 58-60.

Layden, T. 1996. Thrills and spills. *Sports Illustrated*. 12 August, 34-46.

———. 1994. Now for the hard part. *Sports Illustrated.* 6 May, 62-65.

———. 1994. The long road back. *Sports Illustrated.* 23 May, 44-50.

Loehr, J. 1982. *Athletic Excellence.* Denver, CO: Forum.

McCallum, J. 1996. The long haul. *Sports Illustrated.* Olympic Preview. 21 July, 118-122.

Montville, L. 1996. Go Blue! *Sports Illustrated.* 29 July, 40-45.

Oh, S., and D. Falkner. 1985. *A Zen Way of Baseball.* New York, NY: Random House.

Orlick, T. 1990. *In Pursuit of Excellence (2nd ed.).* Champaign, IL: Human Kinetics.

Price, S.L. 1994. Anarchy and Agassi. *Sports Illustrated.* 19 September, 34-36.

Ravizza, K., and T. Hanson. 1995. *Heads Up Baseball.* Indianapolis, IN: Masters Press.

Reilly, R. 1995. Goodness gracious, he's a great ball of fire. *Sports Illustrated.* 27 March, 62-72.

———. 1997. Strokes of genius. *Sports Illustrated.* 21 April, 35-49.

Ryan, J. 1995. *Little Girls in Pretty Boxes.* New York, NY: Doubleday.

Schloegl, I. 1975. *Wisdom of Zen Masters.* New York: New Directions.

Schumacher, J. 1997. Back from oblivion: Hurley—yes, *that* Hurley—is contributing. *The Sacramento Bee.* 8 April, D-1.

Seligman, M.E.P. 1990. *Learned Optimism.* New York, NY: Alfred A. Knopf.

Silverstein, S. 1981. *A Light in the Attic.* New York, NY: HarperCollins Children's Books.

Smith, G. 1996. The tortoise and the hare. *Sports Illustrated.* Olympic Preview. 21 July, 72-85.

Swift, E.M. 1996. Driving Dominique. *Sports Illustrated.* Olympic Preview. 21 July, 86-90.

———. 1996. Profile in courage. *Sports Illustrated.* 5 August, 58-65.

Taylor, J. 1988. Slumpbusting: A Systematic Analysis of Slumps in Sports. *The Sport Psychologist* 2(1):39-48.

Taylor, P. 1997. The rise and fall. *Sports Illustrated.* 21 April, 96-98.

Telander, R. 1995. Purple haze. *Sports Illustrated.* 25 December, 96-110.

Wolff, A. 1996. On the move. *Sports Illustrated.* Olympic Preview. 21 July, 152-158.

Vigeland, C. 1996. *Stalking the Shark: Pressure and Passion on the Pro Golf Tour.* New York, NY: Norton.

INDEX

A

Abbott, Jim, 202
accidents, fear of, 95-96
actions, changing, 125-127
adversity, 224-226
aerobic endurance training, 11
affirmations, 60, 124-125
Agassi, Andre, 20-22
agility training, 10
Ali, Muhammad, 199, 200
anaerobic endurance training, 10-11
Anatomy of an Illness (Cousins), 129
arousal. *See* physiological arousal
associated images, 96
athletes
   learning from, 129-130, 175
   relationship with coaches, 13-14
athletic excellence, 10-11
Atlas, Teddy, 89-90
auditory distractions, 60, 67-68, 72
auditory focus, 59-60, 67-69, 70-71
autogenic training, 251
automatic quality, 6

B

bad habits, ingraining, 137
bad mental strategies, 28-29
Bannister, Roger, 127, 216
Barnett, Gary, 110-111
beliefs. *See also* negative beliefs
   power of, 100-101
   structure of, 104-108
Berra, Yogi, 6, 230, 233
big-enough why, 169-171, 194, 210, 255
Bird, Larry, 63, 202
Blair, Bonnie, 114
Bleier, Rocky, 169-170
body strength training, 10
Boggs, Wade, 87
Boitano, Brian, 149
Bolleteri, Nick, 21
Bowe, Riddick, 76
breathing techniques, 12, 251, 255
Brown, Les, 216

Budd, Zola, 132
burnout, 18-20

C

Calipari, John, 212
catastrophizing, 82
challenge, sense of, 5-6
Chinese female athletes, 220-221
choking, fear as cause, 77-78
Chow, Amy, 207
chronic fatigue, 18
chunking-down strategy, 90-92, 173-174
Churchill, Winston, 216
Clark, Ron, 101
coaches
   belief in athlete, 214
   confidence-instilling role of, 211-213
   consulting with, 14
   effects on performance, 39-41
   failure reactions of, 222
   goal-setting role of, 172-173
   impact of, 13-14
   language choices of, 236
   mental rehearsal assignments by, 138-139, 151
   as slump breakers, 41, 42
   "small-bite" technique for, 92
   using process and outcome goals, 183
collective team consciousness, 86
comfort zones, 93
concentration
   focus of, 33-36, 45-47, 93-94
   narrowing before performance, 62
   on performance, 5
   on place, 52-55
   testing ability for, 69-73
   on time, 48-52
confidence
   enhancing with nickname, 216
   for peak performance, 5
   preparation for, 202-205
   strategies for building, 213-216
   from training environment, 210-213

Connors, Jimmy, 204
control. *See also* uncontrollables
  of eyes and ears, 57-58
  of nerves, 242-244
  before performance, 58-60
  regaining, 30-32
coping imagery, 147-148, 154-158
Cousins, Norman, 129
cues, 56, 64

D
Daggett, Tim, 24, 129, 223
Dare to Dream (Daggett), 129
deadlines, 179-180
defeating fear
  breaking up fear, 90-92
  challenging fear's logic, 94-95
  creating distance from fear, 95-97
  moving toward fear, 89-90
  reframing fear, 92-93
Devers, Gail, 223
dissociated images, 96
distractions
  auditory, 60, 67-68, 72
  identifying, 70-71
  kinesthetic, 72
Dolan, Tom, 200, 201, 213
Dorrance, Anson, 211-212
Douglas, James "Buster," 100-101

E
Earhart, Amelia, 216
ears
  controlling, 57-58
  performance control of, 64-68
  preperformance control of, 59-60,
    60-64
Edge, The (Ferguson), 169, 203
Ellis, Albert, 238
emotions
  actions affecting, 126
  of failure, 228-230
  and mental toughness, 237-238
endurance training, 10-11
enjoyment, 4-5
excellence, key areas of, 10-11
exercises
  Knowing the Road, 226-227
  Resource Room, 251-255
  Discovering That Superperformer
    Inside (SPI), 195-197

experience, changing, 109-113
externalization, 233
external performance cues, 56, 64
eyes
  controlling, 57-58
  performance control of, 64-68
  preperformance control of, 58-60,
    60-64

F
facial expression, and emotions, 126
failure. *See also* success and failure cycles
  emotions of, 228-230
  explaining, 228-235
  as learning experience, 186-187
  mastering, 221-223
  perspective on, 223-227
  responsibility for, 208
false education, fear based on, 85-86
fans
  distractions by, 68
  effects on performance, 39-41
fear. *See also* defeating fear
  recognizing, 81-83
  understanding, 83-88
fear-busting strategies, 84-85
Ferguson, Howard, 169, 203
fight or flight response, 81
flexibility training, 10
focus. *See also* process focus
  of concentration, 45-47
  consistency of, 37-38
  developing focal points, 68-69
  within here and now, 56-57
  in training environment, 210
follow-through, 209
Four-Minute Mile, The (Bannister), 216
fun, 4-5
future, concentration on, 48-52

G
Gable, Dan, 205, 213
gamesmanship, 55
Gilbert, Brad, 21-22
Gilbert, Rob, 23, 89, 241
goals
  focus on, 185-186
  importance of setting, 146-147
  motivational power of, 169-170
  samples of, 191-193
  visibility of, 210

goal-setting principles
  1:Be Sure the Goal Is Yours, 171-173
  2:Break Goal Into Manageable Parts, 173-179
  3:Set Goal Deadlines, 179-180
  4:Use Both Process and Outcome Goals, 180-183
  5:Make Goals Specific, 183-184
  6:Keep Goals Flexible, 184-187
  7:Frame Goals Positively, 187-189
  8:Make Goals Measurable, 189-190
  9:Write Goals Down, 190-191
Gonzales, Pancho, 216
Gwynn, Tony, 79-80

H
habits, 137, 231
Harmon, Butch, 215
Harper, Robert A., 238
head focus, 47
hearing. *See* ears
here and now
  focus within, 56-57
  rule of, 47-55
  staying in, 56-57, 63
Hoch, Scott, 182
Hurley, Bobby, 234-235
Hurst, Maurice, 76-77

I
illogical reasoning, 86-87
imagery, 123-124. *See also* coping imagery; mastery imagery
imagery development
  accuracy of images, 137-139
  introduction to, 136-137
  mental rehearsal techniques for, 140-146
  problem anticipation in, 146
  proper perspective for, 139-140
images, dissociation of, 96
imagination, and fear, 82
impossible, attempting, 112
I Never Had It Made (Robinson), 216
injury, fear of, 76, 77, 84-85
inner movies, 132-134
intermediate goals, 175
internalization, 233
internal performance cues, 56, 64
in-the-experience focus, 46-47
intimidation, 53-54

J
Jansen, Dan, 49, 223
jinxes, 86-87
Johnson, David, 50
Johnson, Michael, 220
Jordan, Eddie, 235
Jordan, Michael, 114, 184, 200, 211
Joyner-Kersee, Jackie, 114

K
Karolyi, Bela, 229
kinesthetic distractions, 72
kinesthetic focus, 68-69, 70-71
kinesthetic sense, *vs.* visual imagery, 143-144
Korellin, Alexander, 202, 204

L
Laird, James, 126
language
  coaches' choice of, 236
  of mental toughness, 235-236
  permanent, 106-107, 114, 115, 232, 235-236
  personal, 233, 235-236
  pervasive, 232-233, 235-236
Learned Optimism (Seligman), 231-233
Lee, Bruce, 124
lemonade strategy, 116-117, 120-121
Lincoln, Abraham, 216
Linnehan, Kim, 108
Live Your Dreams (Brown), 216
long-term goals, 175, 176-179
losing
  expectations of, 86
  fear of, 78, 81
Louganis, Greg, 173
low self-confidence, 12-14

M
mastery imagery, 148-151, 159-163
Mays, Willie, 115-116
McEnroe, John, 55
mechanical mistakes, 12
media, effects on performance, 39-41
mental arena, 11
mental diet, 216
mental game, 3
mental images, power of, 134-136
mental movies, 132-134
mental place, 53-55
mental preparation, 203

mental rehearsal
  definition of, 131
  before performance, 60
  power of, 135
  proper perspective for, 139-140
  techniques of, 144-146
  in vivid detail, 140-144
  when to use, 148, 151
mental strategies
  consistency of, 37-38
  determining, 27-30
mental time zones, 48-52
mental toughness
  ABCs of, 237-238
  composition of, 220-221
  definitions of, 219
  development of, 51
  language of, 235-236
Miller, Shannon, 207
Mills, Billy, 101
Moceanu, Dominique, 207, 229
Montana, Joe, 114, 200
music, as auditory focus, 60

N
Namesnik, Eric, 201
Navratilova, Martina, 2, 216
negative beliefs
  breaking down, 108
  changing actions, 125-127
  changing self-talk, 113-114
  changing the experience, 109-113
  changing time frame, 114
  ignoring experts, 127-128
  reframing, 116-121
negative feelings, 125
negative goals, reframing, 188-189
negative imagery, 132-134
negative self-talk, 116-117, 120-121
negative thoughts, 120-124
nervousness
  controlling, 242-244
  before performance, 245-249
nicknames, 216
Norman, Greg, 188, 228

O
O'Brien, Dan, 50-51
Oerter, Al, 4
Oh, Sadaharu, 2, 129
opponents
  disruptive behavior of, 55

distractions by, 68
optimal arousal, 244, 245-248
optimism, 231
outcome, uncontrollability of, 33
outcome focus, 165, 166
outcome goals, 192, 193
over-arousal
  lowering, 250-251
  signs of, 245-248
overtraining, 18
overuse injuries, 18

P
Parcells, Bill, 76-77
parents
  effects on performance, 39-41
  goal-setting role of, 172-173
  as slump breakers, 41
passion, 4-5
past
  concentration on, 48-52
  successes of, 129
Payton, Gary, 211
peak performance
  here-and-now rule of, 47-55
  mental strategies for, 29
  principles of, 4-6, 222
  review of, 28, 68
perfect practice, 137
performance
  blaming others for, 39-43
  concentration on, 5
  effects of others, 39-43
  peaks and valleys of, 1-2, 25-26
  principles of, 4-6
  relationship to stress, 243 fig. 10.1
  relaxation during, 6
  review of, 27-28
performance awareness, 16-18
performance cues, 56
performance goals, changing, 255
permanent language, 106-107, 114,
  115, 232, 235-236
personal language, 233, 235-236
pervasive language, 232-233, 235-236
pessimism, 231
physical actions, changing, 125-127
physical arena, 10, 17-18
physical condition, 15-16
physical preparation, 202-205
physiological arousal, 242-244, 247-248

place, concentration on, 52-55
positive affirmations, 124-125
possible, belief in, 100
posture, and emotions, 126
preperformance affirmations, 60
preperformance arousal, 249
preperformance control, 58-60
preperformance nervousness, 245-249
preperformance rituals, 60-64, 66-67, 88
present, concentration on, 48-52
prioritizing efforts, 179-180
problem anticipation, 146
process focus, 33, 48, 57, 165-166
process goals, 192-193
progressive muscle relaxation, 251
psychological muscle, 220

Q

questionnaires
   burnout, 19-20
   control, 31-32
   physical, technical, tactical, 17-18
   slump meter, 257-258
Quick, Richard, 11
Quirot, Ana, 220

R

rational emotive therapy, 238
Ravizza, Ken, 59
reading suggestions, 216
rebounding, 11
relaxation
   during performance, 6
   as process focus, 57
   script for, 152-153
resilience, 5
resource room, 251-255
rest, importance of, 18-19
Reyes, Gil, 21
Riddoch, Greg, 79-80
rituals
   development and use of, 216
   before performance, 60-64, 66-67, 88
   superstition based, 87-88
Robinson, Jackie, 216
Rodman, Dennis, 119
Rose, Pete, 230
Ruth, Babe, 239
Ryan, Jim, 128

S

Sampras, Pete, 22
Santana, Rosalind, 212

Sasser, Mackey, 2
Sax, Steve, 2
Schwenk, Trippi, 108
self-blame, 233
self-confidence. *See* confidence
self-fulfilling prophecies, 101-102
self-limiting belief, 104-105
self-talk
   changing, 113-114, 255
   and fear, 94-95
Seligman, Martin, 231-233
setbacks, making temporary, 116-117
Shilstone, Mackie, 76
short-term goals, 175
Slaney, Mary Decker, 132
slump meter, 256-258
slumps
   blaming outside sources for, 24-25
   cycle of, 3
   eliminating causes of, 12-16
   mental strategies for, 29
   nonmental causes of, 9-10, 14-15
   planting seeds of, 26-27
   review of, 27-28, 68
   setting deadlines during, 180
speed training, 10
Sports Slump Busting (Goldberg), 6-7
St. Jean, Gary, 235
Staubach, Roger, 205
strength training, 10
stress
   early-warning signs of, 242-244
   relationship to performance, 243 fig.
      10.1
Strug, Kerri, 229-230
success
   adversity's role in, 224-226
   failure's role in, 222-223
   making permanent, 118-119
   responsibility for, 208
   road to, 167-169, 224-225 fig. 9.1
success and failure cycles, 101-104
Superperformer Inside (SPI) exercise,
   194-197
superstitions, 86-88

T

tactical arena, 11, 17-18
tactical place, 53
teammates, effects on performance, 39-
   41

teams
  collective consciousness of, 86
  rituals of, 61
  sample goals for, 193
technical arena, 11, 17-18
thought habits, 231
thought-stopping techniques, 123-124
Tian Wenhui, 221
time, concentration on, 48-52
time frame, changing, 114
time traveling, 52, 66-67
training
  environment for, 210-213
  key areas of, 10-11
  mental review of, 213
  taking responsibility for, 205-208
Training Soccer Champions (Santana), 212
Tyson, Mike, 89, 100-101

U
uncontrollables
  as competitive edge, 36-39
  mastery of, 32-36
  people as, 39-43
under-arousal, 244, 248-249, 255

V
victory logs, 213-214
videotapes, 16
vignettes
  Agassi, Andre, 20-22
  Barnett, Gary, 110-111
  coach impact, 13-14
  Dolan, Tom, 201
  fear-busting strategies, 84-85
  goal focus, 185-186

Hurley, Bobby, 234-235
  mental rehearsal, 142-143
  mental strategies, 37-38
  O'Brien, Dan, 50-51
  permanent language, 106-107
  physiological arousal, 247-248
  Riddoch, Greg, 79-80
  Strug, Kerri, 229-230
  time traveling, 66-67
vision. *See* eyes
visual distractions, 72
visual focus, 58-60, 68-69, 70-71
visualization
  definition of, 131
  techniques for, 97
Vlasov, Yuri, 149
vulnerabilities, identifying, 65

W
weaknesses
  strengthening, 209-210
  using as strengths, 213
weather, as uncontrollable, 38-39
what-ifs, 82-83, 93-94
Wooden, John, 48
Woods, Earl, 214-215
Woods, Tiger, 214-215

Y
Young, Eric, 209-210

Z
Zen Way of Baseball, A (Oh), 129
Zmelik, Robert, 51
Zmeskal, Kim, 229
zone, being in, 1, 46, 48

ABOUT THE AUTHOR

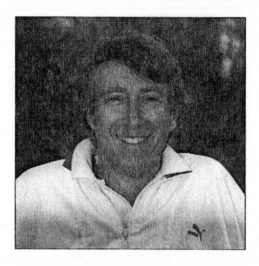

Alan S. Goldberg, EdD, is the director of Competitive Advantage, a sports consulting firm in Amherst, Massachusetts. A practicing sport psychology consultant since 1983, he has worked with hundreds of coaches and slumping athletes and teams across a wide variety of sports, competition levels, and ages. He also has gained a unique perspective on developing mental toughness as a professional tennis instructor for more than 22 years and as a former number one singles player and conference champion as a student at the University of Massachusetts.

Dr. Goldberg is a nationally known expert in the field of applied sport psychology and maintains an extensive speaking schedule. He has written articles for numerous national publications and has published five workbooks and 10 audiocassette programs on mental training techniques. In addition to working with amateur and professional athletes and coaches, Dr. Goldberg is a regular speaker at the U.S. Olympic Training Center in Colorado Springs.

Dr. Goldberg lives in Amherst, Massachusetts, with his wife, Renee, and two daughters, Sara and Julee. He enjoys karate, sports with his children, and the beach.

Printed in the United States
30456LVS00005B/106-162

9 781595 261014